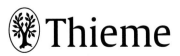

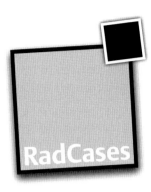

RadCases Musculoskeletal Radiology
Second Edition

Edited by

Glenn M. Garcia, MD
The Robert N. Cooley Executive Vice Chairman of
  Radiology
Associate Professor and Director of Musculoskeletal
  Radiology
University of Texas Medical Branch
Galveston, Texas

Series Editors

Jonathan M. Lorenz, MD, FSIR
Professor of Radiology
Section of Interventional Radiology
The University of Chicago
Chicago, Illinois

Hector Ferral, MD
Senior Medical Educator
NorthShore University HealthSystem
Evanston, Illinois

290 illustrations

Thieme
New York • Stuttgart • Delhi • Rio de Janeiro

Executive Editor: William Lamsback
Managing Editor: J. Owen Zurhellen IV
Associate Managing Editor: Kenneth Schubach
Director, Editorial Services: Mary Jo Casey
Production Editor: Teresa Exley, Absolute Service, Inc.
Editorial Director: Sue Hodgson
International Production Director: Andreas Schabert
International Marketing Director: Fiona Henderson
International Sales Director: Louisa Turrell
Director of Institutional Sales: Adam Bernacki
Senior Vice President and Chief Operating Officer:
    Sarah Vanderbilt
President: Brian D. Scanlan
Printer: Sheridan Books

Library of Congress Cataloging-in-Publication Data

Names: Garcia, Glenn M., editor.
Title: RadCases musculoskeletal radiology / edited by
    Glenn M. Garcia.
Other titles: Musculoskeletal radiology (Garcia)
Description: Second edition. | New York : Thieme, [2018] | Series:
    RadCases | Preceded by Musculoskeletal radiology / edited by
    Glenn M. Garcia. c2010. | Includes bibliographical references
    and index. | Description based on print version record and CIP
    data provided by publisher; resource not viewed.
Identifiers: LCCN 2017031959 (print) | LCCN 2017033855
    (ebook) | ISBN 9781626232457 | ISBN 9781626232440 |
    ISBN 9781626232457 (ebook)
Subjects: | MESH: Musculoskeletal Diseases--diagnostic imaging |
    Radiography | Musculoskeletal System--diagnostic imaging |
    Diagnosis, Differential | Diagnostic Imaging--methods | Case
    Reports
Classification: LCC RC925.7 (ebook) | LCC RC925.7 (print) | NLM
    WE 141 | DDC 616.7/07548--dc23
LC record available at https://lccn.loc.gov/2017031959

Copyright © 2018 by Thieme Medical Publishers, Inc.
Thieme Publishers New York
333 Seventh Avenue, New York, NY 10001 USA
+1 800 782 3488, customerservice@thieme.com

Thieme Publishers Stuttgart
Rüdigerstrasse 14, 70469 Stuttgart, Germany
+49 [0]711 8931 421, customerservice@thieme.de

Thieme Publishers Delhi
A-12, Second Floor, Sector-2, Noida-201301
Uttar Pradesh, India
+91 120 45 566 00, customerservice@thieme.in

Thieme Publishers Rio de Janeiro, Thieme Publicações Ltda.
Edifício Rodolpho de Paoli, 25º andar
Av. Nilo Peçanha, 50 – Sala 2508,
Rio de Janeiro 20020-906 Brasil
+55 21 3172-2297/+55 21 3172-1896

Cover design: Thieme Publishing Group
Typesetting by Absolute Service, Inc.

Printed in the United States by Sheridan Books
5 4 3 2 1

ISBN 978-1-62623-244-0

Also available as an e-book:
eISBN 978-1-62623-245-7

Important note: Medicine is an ever-changing science undergoing continual development. Research and clinical experience are continually expanding our knowledge, in particular our knowledge of proper treatment and drug therapy. Insofar as this book mentions any dosage or application, readers may rest assured that the authors, editors, and publishers have made every effort to ensure that such references are in accordance with **the state of knowledge at the time of production of the book**.

Nevertheless, this does not involve, imply, or express any guarantee or responsibility on the part of the publishers in respect to any dosage instructions and forms of applications stated in the book. **Every user is requested to examine carefully** the manufacturers' leaflets accompanying each drug and to check, if necessary in consultation with a physician or specialist, whether the dosage schedules mentioned therein or the contraindications stated by the manufacturers differ from the statements made in the present book. Such examination is particularly important with drugs that are either rarely used or have been newly released on the market. Every dosage schedule or every form of application used is entirely at the user's own risk and responsibility. The authors and publishers request every user to report to the publishers any discrepancies or inaccuracies noticed. If errors in this work are found after publication, errata will be posted at www.thieme.com on the product description page.

Some of the product names, patents, and registered designs referred to in this book are in fact registered trademarks or proprietary names even though specific reference to this fact is not always made in the text. Therefore, the appearance of a name without designation as proprietary is not to be construed as a representation by the publisher that it is in the public domain.

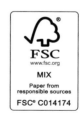

Dedicated to Kelley and Claire!

Series Preface

As enthusiastic partners in radiology education, we continue our mission to ease the exhaustion and frustration shared by residents and the families of residents engaged in radiology training! In launching the second edition of the RadCases series, our intent is to expand rather than replace this already rich study experience that has been tried, tested, and popularized by residents around the world. In each subspecialty edition, we serve up 100 new, carefully chosen cases to raise the bar in our effort to assist residents in tackling the daunting task of assimilating massive amounts of information. RadCases second edition primes and expands on concepts found in the first edition with important variations on prior cases, updated diagnostic and management strategies, and new pathological entities. Our continuing goal is to combine the popularity and portability of printed books with the adaptability, exceptional quality, and interactive features of an electronic case–based format. The new cases will be added to the existing electronic database to enrich the interactive environment of high-quality images that allows residents to arrange study sessions, quickly extract and master information, and prepare for theme-based radiology conferences.

We owe a debt of gratitude to our own residents and to the many radiology trainees who have helped us create, adapt, and improve the format and content of RadCases by weighing in with suggestions for new cases, functions, and formatting. Back by popular demand is the concise, point-by-point presentation of the Essential Facts of each case in an easy-to-read bulleted format, and a short, critical differential starting with the actual diagnosis. This approach is easy on exhausted eyes and encourages repeated priming of important information during quick reviews, a process we believe is critical to radiology education. New since the prior edition is the addition of a question-and-answer section for each case to reinforce key concepts.

The intent of the printed books is to encourage repeated priming in the use of critical information by providing a portable group of exceptional core cases to master. Unlike the authors of other case-based radiology review books, we removed the guesswork by providing clear annotations and descriptions for all images. In our opinion, there is nothing worse than being unable to locate a subtle finding on a poorly reproduced image even after one knows the final diagnosis.

The electronic cases expand on the printed book and provide a comprehensive review of the entire specialty. Thousands of cases are strategically designed to increase the resident's knowledge by providing exposure to a spectrum of case examples—from basic to advanced—and by exploring "Aunt Minnie's," unusual diagnoses, and variability within a single diagnosis. The search engine allows the resident to create individualized daily study lists that are not limited by factors such as radiology subsection. For example, tailor today's study list to cases involving tuberculosis and include cases in every subspecialty and every system of the body. Or study only thoracic cases, including those with links to cardiology, nuclear medicine, and pediatrics. Or study only musculoskeletal cases. The choice is yours.

As enthusiastic partners in this project, we started small and, with the encouragement, talent, and guidance of Timothy Hiscock and William Lamsback at Thieme Publishers, we have further raised the bar in our effort to assist residents in tackling the daunting task of assimilating massive amounts of information. We are passionate about continuing this journey and will continue to expand the series, adapt cases based on direct feedback from residents, and increase the features intended for board review and self-assessment. First and foremost, we thank our medical students, residents, and fellows for allowing us the privilege to participate in their educational journey.

Jonathan M. Lorenz, MD, FSIR
Hector Ferral, MD

Preface

This second edition of RadCases provides the most updated information regarding all facets of musculoskeletal imaging. Multimodality imaging of a variety of musculoskeletal conditions intermixed with physics principles, imaging artifacts, and common anatomic variants are presented. Cases include realistic clinical presentations, reasonable differential diagnoses, and case summaries with updated references.

This second edition was developed to further serve radiologists of all skill levels. This includes radiology residents in training; radiologists seeking board certification/maintenance of certification; or seasoned, clinically active radiologists seeking fundamental information in musculoskeletal imaging.

Case 1

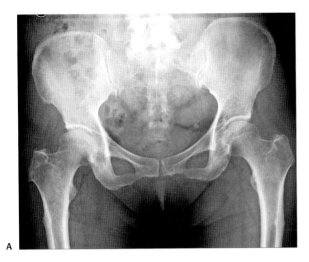

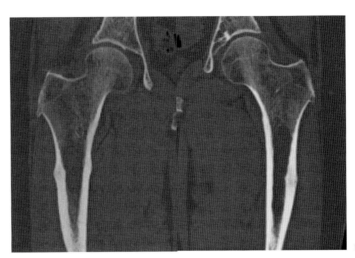

A   B

■ Clinical Presentation

An elderly female patient presents with chronic hip pain and osteoporosis on bisphosphonate therapy.

■ Imaging Findings

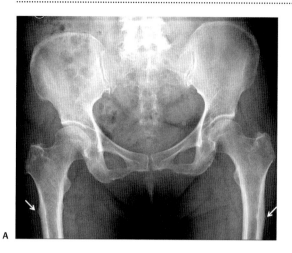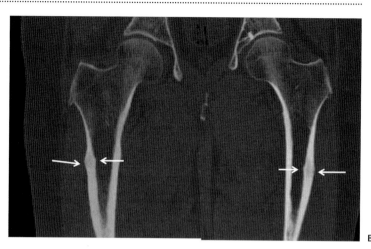

A   B

(A) Pelvic radiograph demonstrates lateral subtrochanteric femoral cortical thickening (*arrows*). **(B)** Coronal reconstructed CT scan demonstrates pointing or spiking of the cortices (*arrows*) with an incomplete fracture on the left.

■ Differential Diagnosis

- ***Bisphosphonate-related femoral fractures:*** Insufficiency fractures associated with long-term bisphosphonate use commonly occurring along the proximal lateral femoral cortices.
- *Linea aspera:* Normal bony ridge along the posterior mid/proximal femur serving as the attachment site for the adductor musculature.

■ Essential Facts

- Bisphosphonate-related femoral fractures are considered insufficiency fractures.
- The typical patient is a postmenopausal elderly female with a history of long-term bisphosphonate use for osteoporosis.
- These fractures frequently involve the lateral femoral cortex.
- Findings are frequently superimposed upon an osteopenic skeleton.
- Radiographs and CT scans reveal beaking or pointing of the cortices along the fracture margins secondary to the healing process.

■ Other Imaging Findings

- Radionuclide bone scan will show increased radiotracer uptake at the fracture sites.

✓ Pearls and ✗ Pitfalls

- ✓ Greater than 50% of these fractures are bilateral.
- ✓ Greater than 50% of these fractures occur along the femoral diaphysis within 5 cm of the lesser trochanter.
- ✗ Given the subtrochanteric location of these fractures, routine hip and knee radiographs may exclude the pathology from the field of view. Therefore, femoral radiographs may be necessary to achieve the diagnosis.

Case 2

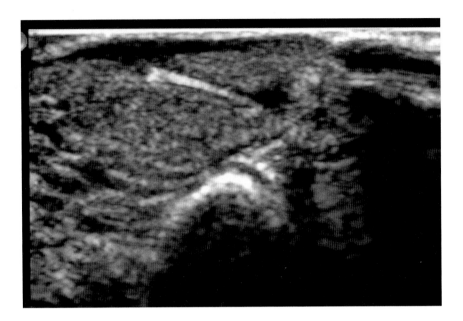

■ Clinical Presentation

A 40-year-old male with soft tissue swelling of the distal ring finger with remote history of penetrating injury.

■ **Imaging Findings**

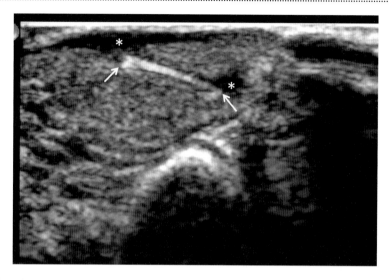

Ultrasound image obtained along the volar aspect of the distal ring finger demonstrates a linear echogenic foreign body (*arrows*) within the subcutaneous fat. Sonolucent fluid (*asterisks*) is seen along the proximal and distal margins of this structure.

■ **Differential Diagnosis**

- ***Echogenic linear foreign body:*** An echogenic, linear, non-anatomic foreign structure with surrounding fluid in a patient presenting with a history of penetrating injury is diagnostic of a foreign body.
- *Subcutaneous abscess:* A focal hypoechoic or anechoic heterogeneous fluid collection containing irregular or circumscribed borders.

■ **Essential Facts**

- Penetrating injuries with a retained foreign body represent a common cause for emergency room visits.
- Ultrasound imaging enables detection of a host of foreign bodies that include splinters, glass, plastic, and metal.
- The most common retained foreign bodies include wood, glass, and metal.
- When performing the exam, the area of interest should be imaged in longitudinal and transverse planes with utilization of a 7.5- to 10-MHz transducer.
- Characteristic ultrasound features of a foreign body include a linear echogenic structure with or without acoustic shadowing.
- A surrounding hypoechoic rim may be present around foreign bodies implanted > 24 hours.

- Reportable features should include the depth of the foreign body and the proximity of the foreign body to adjacent joints, tendon sheaths, nerves, or vascular structures.
- Assessment for adjacent fluid collections is essential.
- Correlation with radiographs is essential.

✓ **Pearls and ✗ Pitfalls**

- ✓ All superficial foreign bodies are echogenic and potentially detectable on ultrasound.
- ✓ Dystrophic soft tissue calcifications may result in a false-positive finding with ultrasound imaging.
- ✗ Obscuration of foreign bodies may occur secondary to shadowing from adjacent soft tissue gas or cortical bone.

Case 3

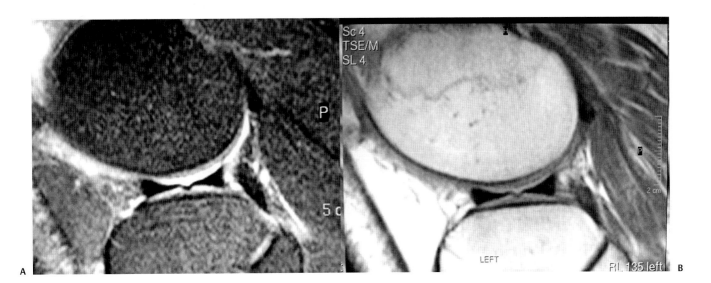

■ Clinical Presentation

A patient presents with swelling and pain.

■ **Imaging Findings**

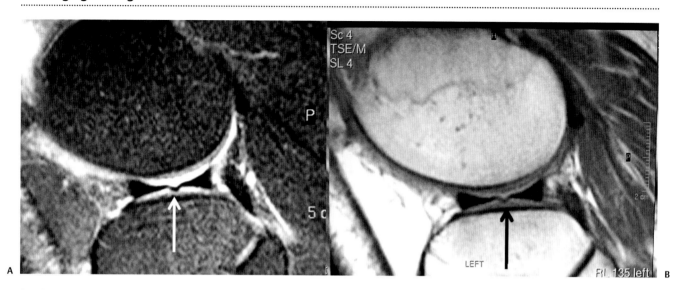

(A, B) Sagittal fluid-sensitive and fat-sensitive MR sequences through the lateral meniscus demonstrate wrinkling or flouncing along the body of the meniscus (*arrows*).

■ **Differential Diagnosis**

- ***Meniscal flounce:*** A transient positional waviness assumed by the meniscus.
- *Meniscal tear:* Internal T2 signal derangement within a meniscus that exhibits extension to an articular surface.

■ **Essential Facts**

- The meniscal flounce is related to transient positional distortion which is dependent on flexion and external rotation.
- Incidence on MRI ranges from 0.1 to 6%.
- Typically described as a normal variant.

✓ **Pearls and ✗ Pitfalls**

- ✓ Meniscal flounce is more common in the medial meniscus.
- ✗ Some meniscal tears may result in a flouncelike appearance.

Case 4

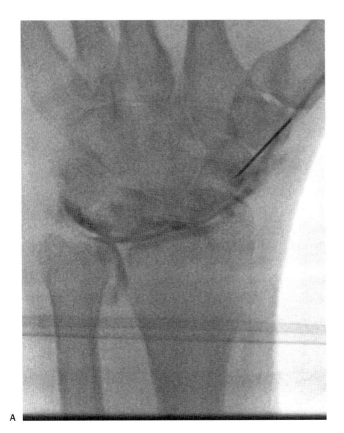

A

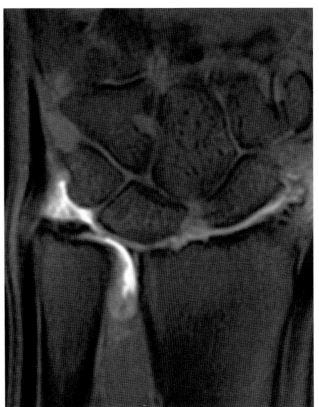

B

■ Clinical Presentation

A middle-aged female patient presents with ulnar-sided wrist pain and an audible click.

■ Imaging Findings

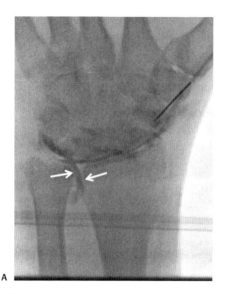 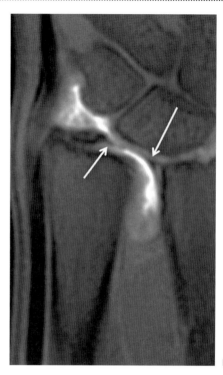

(A) A fluoroscopic spot film from a single-compartment radiocarpal wrist arthrogram injection displays contrast extravasation (*arrows*) into the distal radial ulnar joint (DRUJ). **(B)** A coronal T1 fat-suppressed MR arthrogram through the DRUJ demonstrates absence of the central membranous segment of the triangular fibrocartilage (TFC). There is peripheral displacement (*arrows*) of the residual TFC.

■ Differential Diagnosis

• ***Tear of the triangular fibrocartilage:*** A mechanical or degenerative process causing disruption of the triangular fibrocartilage (TFC). Arthrography demonstrates free passage of contrast between the radiocarpal and distal radial ulnar joints. MRI findings consistent with a tear include disruption of this low-signal cartilaginous disk with hyperintense T2 fluid signal intensity.

■ Essential Facts

• The TFC is a semicircular biconcave fibrocartilaginous structure that acts as a stabilizer and shock absorber for the DRUJ and ulnar carpal joints. The central portion of the TFC is thinner than the periphery and is referred to as the *membranous segment*.
• The TFC is primarily anchored to the medial radius and ulnar styloid.
• TFC tears are best evaluated with MR arthrography following fluoroscopic wrist arthrography.

• The injection solution is composed of 1 part gadolinium to 200 parts saline and iodinated contrast.
• For radiocarpal injections, the needle tip should be placed at the mid-scaphoid or proximal pole just lateral to the scapholunate interval.
• Extension of contrast from the radiocarpal joint into the DRUJ on radiographs is an indication of a TFC tear.
• TFC tears may be degenerative or traumatic.

✓ Pearls and ✗ Pitfalls

✓ Younger patients are more prone to traumatic TFC tears.
✓ Radiographs with ulnar positive variance and cystic changes in the lunate (ulnar impaction) are highly associated with TFC tears.
✓ Fractures through the base of the ulnar styloid are likely to cause detachment of the TFC from the ulna.
✗ Patients older than ~35 to 40 years of age will frequently exhibit asymptomatic membranous perforations through the TFC, emphasizing the importance of clinical presentation.

Case 5

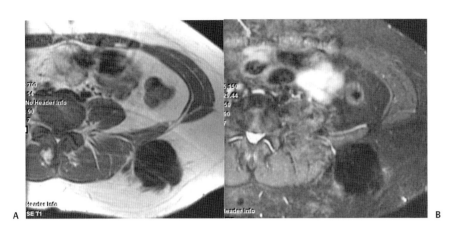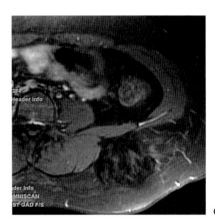

A   SE T1   B   C

■ **Clinical Presentation**
....

A 35-year-old female patient presents with a slowly enlarging left flank mass.

■ Imaging Findings

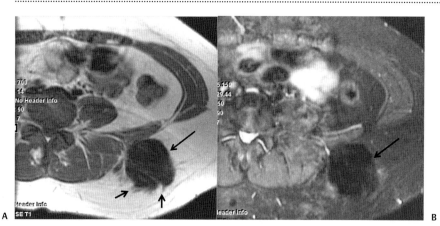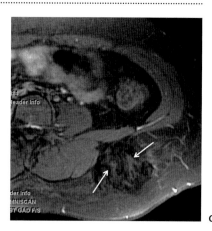

(A, B) Axial fat-sensitive and fluid-sensitive MR images reveal a low-signal solid subcutaneous mass (*long arrows*) abutting the left paraspinal and quadratus lumborum muscular fascia. Note the posterior spiculated infiltrative margins extending into the subcutaneous fat (*short arrows*). **(C)** Post-contrast axial T1 fat-suppressed MR image demonstrates internal heterogeneous irregular enhancement (*arrows*).

■ **Differential Diagnosis**

- *Desmoid tumor:* Benign, locally aggressive fibrous neoplasm frequently seen in females.
- *Nodular fasciitis:* Benign fibrous lesion commonly seen within the distal upper extremities.
- *Myositis ossificans:* A posttraumatic ossified lesion positioned within the musculature.

■ **Essential Facts**

- Desmoid tumor is a neoplastic lesion typically composed of an abundance of fibrous tissue/collagen.
- Abdominal and extra-abdominal desmoid variants exist, with intra-abdominal desmoids frequently associated with Gardner's syndrome.
- Peak incidence of extra-abdominal desmoids is 25 to 35 years of age; seen with a 2:1 female-to-male ratio.
- The lesions originate from abdominal and extra-abdominal connective tissue, fascia, aponeuroses, and musculature.

- These are slow-growing lesions.
- 10% of cases may be multicentric.
- MRI demonstrates decreased T1 and T2 signal with spiculated infiltrative margins.

■ **Other Imaging Findings**

- Three-phase radionuclide bone scan may reveal uptake within these lesions on blood pool and delayed static images.

✓ **Pearls and** ✗ **Pitfalls**

✓ The most common location for extra-abdominal desmoids includes the proximal upper extremities, chest wall, flank, and the head/neck area.
✗ These lesions may show internal T2 signal increase inversely proportional to the organized fibrous/collagen content, potentially complicating the diagnosis.

Case 6

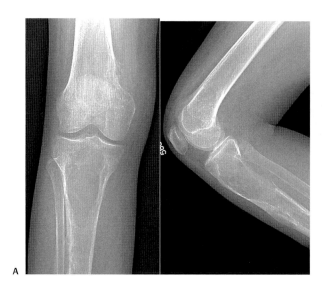

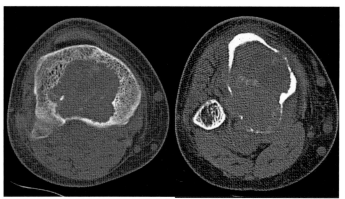

A

B

■ Clinical Presentation

A 24-year-old female patient presents with chronic metabolic derangement.

■ Further Work-up

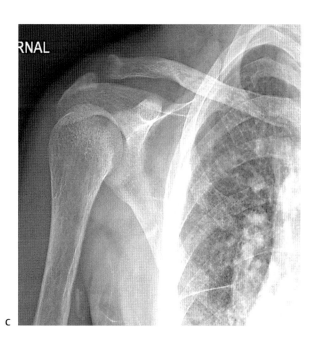

C

■ **Imaging Findings**

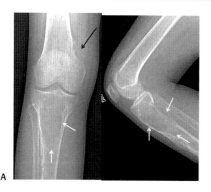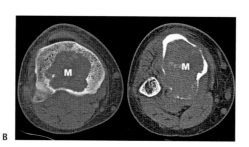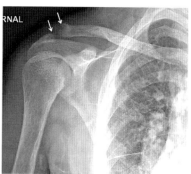

(A) Tibia radiographs demonstrate a lytic expansile lesion (*white arrows*) replacing the proximal tibia with smooth margins, thinning of the cortices, and faint internal calcifications. A separate eccentric distal medial femoral supracondylar lesion is seen (*black arrow*). Diffuse osteopenia is present. **(B)** Axial CT images through the tibial lesion (*M*) demonstrate replacement of the trabeculae with a hypodense lesion containing faint internal calcifications. There is thinning, ballooning, and fenestration of the cortices, with no soft tissue mass seen. **(C)** Shoulder radiograph displays erosions (*arrows*) along the articular margins of the acromioclavicular joint.

■ **Differential Diagnosis**

• **Renal osteodystrophy with multicentric brown tumor formation:** Metabolic bone disease resulting from chronic renal disease causing diffuse osteopenia, acromioclavicular (AC) joint erosions, and multifocal lytic lesions.
• *Metastases:* Lytic osseous lesions of variable sizes related to a primary tumor are characteristic radiographic findings for metastases. However, this patient's younger age combined with osteopenia, periarticular AC joint erosions, and history of "metabolic derangement" do not favor this diagnosis.
• *Multiple myeloma:* A primary bone marrow plasma cell dyscrasia. Although diffuse osteopenia and lytic osseous lesions may be seen in multiple myeloma, the variable-sized bony lesions and the patient's youth argue against this diagnosis.

■ **Essential Facts**

• Renal osteodystrophy results from retention of phosphate and decreased vitamin D synthesis causing parathyroid hormone elevation.
• Parathyroid hormone elevation may lead to subchondral, subligamentous, subtendinous, periarticular, subperiosteal, trabecular, and endosteal bone resorption.

• Large lytic lesions composed of blood products, fibrous tissue, and osteoclasts may arise in the long and flat bones referred to as *brown tumors.* These tumors are more frequently seen with primary hyperparathyroidism.
• This diagnosis is commonly seen as a result of diabetic nephropathy, accounting for the descriptive diagnosis of renal osteodystrophy.

■ **Other Imaging Findings**

• Bone scintigraphy may show diffuse skeletal radiotracer uptake and diminished activity within the kidneys/soft tissues consistent with a superscan.

✓ **Pearls and ✗ Pitfalls**

✓ Acroosteolysis and radial-sided resorption along the middle phalanges of the second and third digits are diagnostic of this disease process.
✗ Exclusion of metastasis and myeloma may be particularly difficult in older patients with renal osteodystrophy, given the overlap of imaging findings.

Case 7

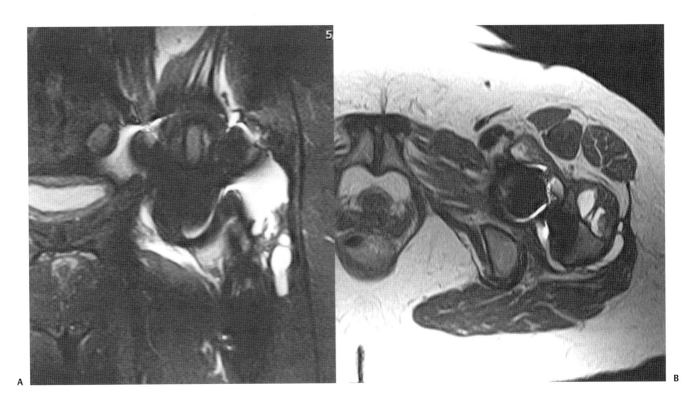

■ Clinical Presentation

A 53-year-old female patient presents with a history of metal-on-metal (MOM) left total hip arthroplasty (THA) with pain and fullness.

■ **Imaging Findings**

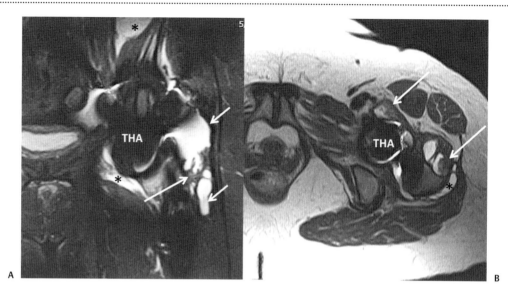

(A, B) Coronal short tau inversion recovery (STIR) and axial T2-weighted MR images of the left hip demonstrate cystic (*short arrows*) and solid (*long arrows*) soft tissue masses surrounding susceptibility artifact from a MOM THA. Portions of the fluid dissect beyond the constraints of the joint capsule (*asterisk*). A low signal rim surrounds this cystic and solid mass lesion.

■ **Differential Diagnosis**

- ***Pseudotumor:*** Expansile cystic and solid lesion associated with MOM THAs which may extend from the hip joint capsule into the surrounding tissues.
- *Reactive joint effusion/synovitis:* Fluid and synovial thickening confined to the joint capsule is characteristic of this finding.
- *Hematoma:* Mixed increased T1/T2 signal intensity fluid collection centered within or adjacent to the joint capsule consistent with blood products.

■ **Essential Facts**

- *Pseudotumor* is a term associated with adverse reaction to metal debris or adverse local tissue reaction described in the context of THA utilizing MOM components.
- The pathophysiology most likely relates to metallic wear particles/debris and reactive tissue inflammation from metal ions and corrosion products related to MOM THA components.
- This process is related to a range of inflammatory reactions thought to be driven by an immune response to metallic wear particles resembling a type IV immune hypersensitivity reaction.
- An MR classification scheme exists characterizing lesion size, capsular rupture, cystic and solid synovial patterns, and synovial thickening in an effort to predict intraoperative tissue damage and extent of inflammation.

- A low T1/T2 signal rim is often seen surrounding this cystic and solid lesion.
- Tissue necrosis may occur, resulting in extension of joint fluid beyond the confines of the joint capsule with extension into adjacent bursae.
- Adjacent muscle and tendon tears with muscle atrophy may occur.

■ **Other Imaging Findings**

- CT scan may demonstrate lobulated mixed fluid and soft tissue density components along the course of the THA components.

✓ **Pearls and ✕ Pitfalls**

- ✓ MRI findings of synovial thickening of > 7 mm correlates with a severe soft tissue inflammatory reaction.
- ✓ MRI findings of capsular dehiscence and a mixed appearance of synovitis and extra-capsular synovial herniation are strongly correlated with intraoperative tissue damage.
- ✕ Early changes of this disease process may be obscured by susceptibility artifact from hardware components if metal artifact reduction MRI sequences are not utilized.

Case 8

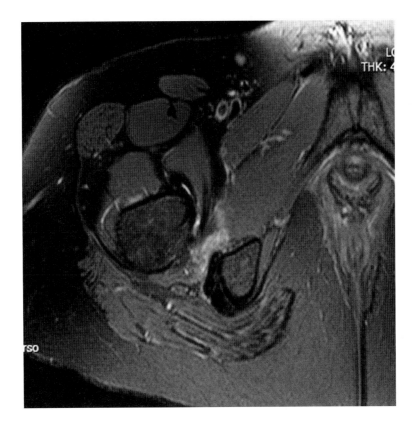

■ Clinical Presentation

A 37-year-old female patient presents with posterior right hip pain, without a history of trauma.

■ **Imaging Findings**

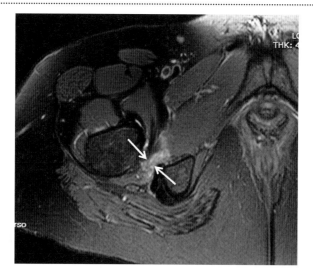

Axial fluid-sensitive MR image through the right hip demonstrates moderate central quadratus femoris muscle edema (*arrows*) without muscle fiber interruption.

■ **Differential Diagnosis**

• ***Ischiofemoral impingement:*** An extra-articular impingement disorder seen about the hip. Central focal quadratus femoris muscle belly edema in a female presenting with posterior right hip pain without antecedent trauma favors this diagnosis.
• *Denervation edema:* A process causing geographic muscle edema related to the early stages of denervation.
• *Exercise-induced edema:* Global muscle edema associated with rigorous exercise.

■ **Essential Facts**

• Ischiofemoral impingement is described as crowding of the fibers of the quadratus femoris muscle belly between the ischium and/or hamstring tendons and the posteromedial femur.
• This narrowing may be congenital or acquired.
• This diagnosis is typically seen in the middle-aged or older female who presents with posterior hip or gluteal pain.
• This diagnosis is best made on axial fluid-sensitive MR images.
• A mixture of edema and/or fatty atrophy may occur, depending on the chronicity and severity.
• A correlation may exist with ischiofemoral impingement and narrowing of the ischiofemoral space (distance between the lateral cortex of the ischial tuberosity and medial cortex of the lesser trochanter) of 13 mm or less on axial images.

• A correlation may exist with ischiofemoral impingement and narrowing of the quadratus femoris space (distance between the superior and lateral surface of the hamstring tendon and the posterior and medial surface of the iliopsoas tendon or lesser trochanter) of 7 mm or less on axial images.

■ **Other Imaging Findings**

• Findings on CT scan may show fatty infiltration of the quadratus femoris musculature in the more chronic phase of this disease.

✓ **Pearls and ✗ Pitfalls**

✓ Quadratus femoris muscle edema associated with ischiofemoral impingement is typically centered within the central muscle belly. This is opposed to the musculotendinous edema seen from muscle strains and the global edema with denervation edema.
✓ Ischiofemoral impingement may be bilateral in up to 40% of patients.
✗ Measurements for the ischiofemoral and quadratus femoris spaces may be overestimated with external rotation of the hips.

Case 9

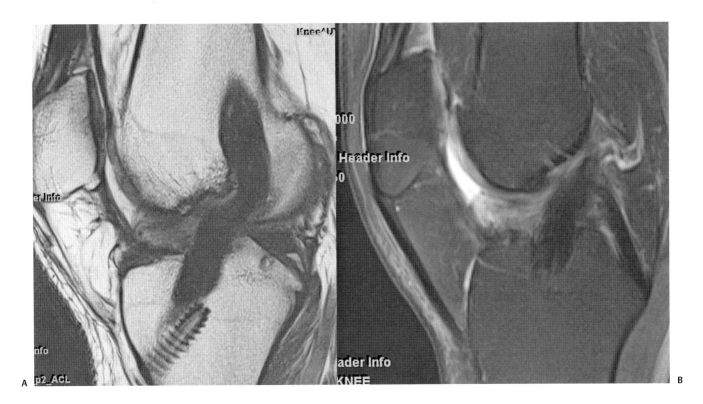

■ Clinical Presentation

A patient presents with a history of knee surgery with block to extension.

■ Imaging Findings

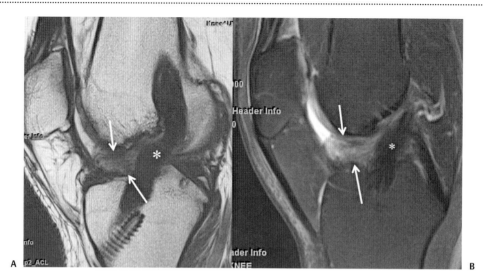

A   B

(A, B) Sagittal proton density and T2-weighted fat saturation MR images demonstrate an intermediate signal intensity nodule (*arrows*) within the intercondylar notch intimately associated with the anterior distal fibers of an anterior cruciate ligament graft (*asterisk*).

■ Differential Diagnosis

• ***Cyclops lesion-lobulated fibrous tissue formation:***
  Typically related to anterior cruciate ligament (ACL)
  surgery in which the fibrous mass adheres to the anterior
  and distal ACL graft fibers demonstrating intermediate
  MR signal intensity.
• *Focal pigmented villonodular synovitis:* A focal synovial-
  based neoplastic process producing an intracapsular
  lobulated lesion which may exhibit blooming artifact on
  MRI secondary to hemosiderin accumulation.

■ Essential Facts

• A cyclops lesion is a firm, fairly noncompressible lesion
  composed of synovial tissue, fibrosis, ACL tissue, and
  bone debris.
• Patients typically present with a block to extension
  secondary to mass effect from the lesion abutting the
  anterior intercondylar notch.

• This lesion may arise from a combination of residual torn
  ACL tissue, ACL graft tissue, infrapatellar fatty metaplasia,
  intercondylar fibrosis, and/or microtrauma.
• This lesion typically contains intermediate signal
  intensity on T2-weighted and proton density images.
• Presentation is on average 4 months after ACL surgery.
• Cure is via arthroscopic resection.

✓ Pearls and ✗ Pitfalls

✓ A minority of cyclops lesions may occur in the absence
  of surgery secondary to remote subclinical partial or
  complete ACL tears.
✗ A cyclopoid lesion/scar may occur adjacent to the ACL,
  which should not be confused with a cyclops lesion.
  This type of lesion is compressible and does not cause
  the characteristic block to extension.

Case 10

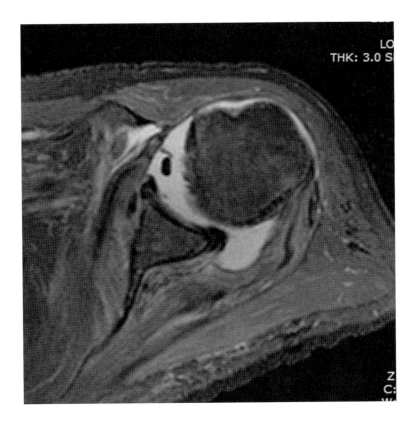

■ Clinical Presentation

A patient presents with left arm weakness and pain.

■ **Imaging Findings**

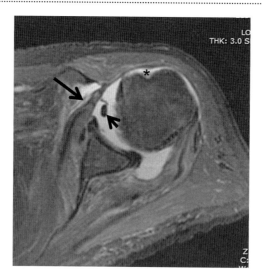

Axial fluid-sensitive MR imaging through the left shoulder demonstrates a full-thickness retracted tear through the subscapularis tendon (*long arrow*). Medial intra-articular biceps tendon dislocation (*short arrow*) is demonstrated. Also displayed is a large-sized joint effusion with posterior humeral head subluxation and an empty biceps sulcus (*asterisk*).

■ **Differential Diagnosis**

• ***Medial biceps tendon dislocation with subscapularis tendon tear:*** Uncovering of the biceps sulcus roof secondary to a full-thickness rupture of the subscapularis tendon allowing for medial biceps tendon dislocation and an empty biceps sulcus is consistent with this diagnosis.
• *Buford complex:* A variant consisting of a hypertrophied middle glenohumeral ligament with paucity of anterior superior labral tissue.

■ **Essential Facts**

• The biceps tendon is composed of a long and a short head, with the long head originating from the superior glenoid tubercle and the short head originating from the coracoid process. The tendon inserts distally at the level of the radial tuberosity.
• The subscapularis tendon inserts onto the lesser tuberosity of the humerus with lateral extension of fibers that insert into the transverse humeral ligament, which helps to secure the biceps tendon within the biceps sulcus.

• Full-thickness disruption of the subscapularis tendon fibers superiorly allows medial biceps tendon dislocation between the humeral head and glenoid.
• Biceps tendon dislocations can be identified medial to the bicipital groove, most clearly seen on axial MR images.
• Tendon dislocation may also occur anterior to the subscapularis tendon or within the substance of the subscapularis tendon.

✓ **Pearls and ✗ Pitfalls**

✓ Marked fatty replacement of the subscapularis musculature related to a chronic subscapularis tendon tear should raise suspicion for biceps tendon subluxation/dislocation.
✗ Absence of a joint effusion and internal rotation of the glenohumeral joint may limit the ability to diagnose a biceps tendon dislocation.

Case 11

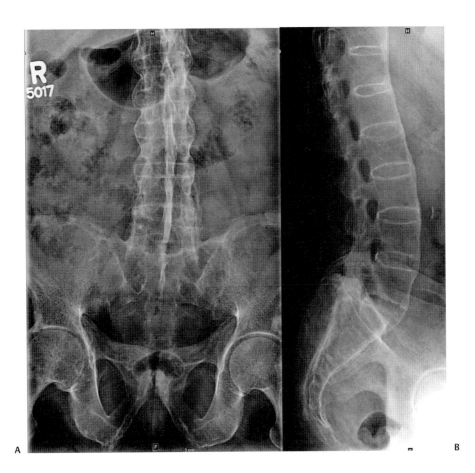

A   B

■ Clinical Presentation

A young adult Latino male presents with a long-standing history of low back pain.

■ Imaging Findings

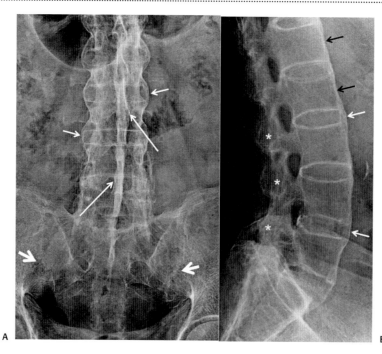

(A, B) Frontal and lateral radiographs of the lumbar spine demonstrate bilateral sacroiliac joint fusion (*thick white arrows*). The lateral view displays squaring of the anterior lumbar vertebral body cortices (*short black arrows*) related to new bone formation. Syndesmophyte formation (*short white arrows*) bridges the vertebral bodies, causing a "bamboo spine" on the frontal radiograph. Dense ossification of the interspinous ligament (*long white arrows*) causes a "dagger" sign. Osseous fusion through the facet joints (*asterisks*) is seen.

■ Differential Diagnosis

- ***Ankylosing spondylitis (AS):*** A seronegative spondyloarthropathy causing bilateral sacroiliac (SI) joint and articular facet fusion with vertebral body squaring and diffuse, symmetric syndesmophyte formation.
- *Diffuse idiopathic skeletal hyperostosis (DISH):* A degenerative process resulting in bulky paravertebral ossification commonly seen in older adults.
- *Psoriatic arthritis:* A seronegative spondyloarthropathy producing thick irregular paravertebral ossification with asymmetric SI joint erosive changes.

■ Essential Facts

- AS is a chronic inflammatory arthritic condition referred to as a seronegative (rheumatoid factor negative) spondyloarthropathy.
- Many patients are HLA-B27 positive, suggesting a hereditary component.
- This condition is common in young men between the ages of 15 and 35 years and primarily affects the axial skeleton synovial/cartilaginous joints and entheses.
- Erosive changes are followed by bone formation with eventual osseous fusion.
- Radiographic changes include symmetric syndesmophyte formation along the spine creating the appearance of a "bamboo spine."

- Syndesmophyte formation across the interspinous ligament of the spinous processes results in the "dagger" sign on frontal spinal radiographs.
- Cyclical bone production along the anterior vertebral body cortices results in vertebral body squaring, best displayed on lateral lumbar spine radiographs.
- Sacroiliitis is typically symmetric, resulting in eventual ankylosis.

■ Other Imaging Findings

- Nuclear medicine bone scan exhibits symmetric increased radioisotope uptake at the SI joints.

✓ Pearls and ✗ Pitfalls

- ✓ SI joint sclerosis and erosions typically represent the first manifestation of this disease process and are bilateral and symmetric.
- ✓ Syndesmophyte formation typically originates at the thoracolumbar junction.
- ✗ The radiographic appearance of AS may be identical to the skeletal changes caused by inflammatory bowel disease and Crohn's disease.

Case 12

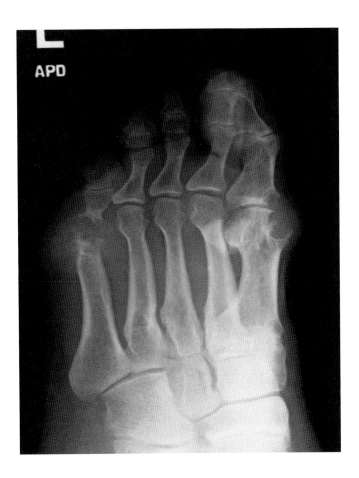

■ Clinical Presentation

A 65-year-old male presents with foot pain.

■ Imaging Findings

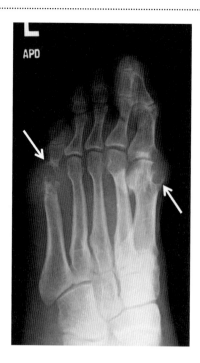

Oblique radiograph of the foot demonstrates fifth metatarsophalangeal (MTP) joint periarticular erosions. Periarticular erosive changes also affect the medial first MTP joint. Overhanging edges (*arrows*) are seen about these erosive margins. No osteopenia is present.

■ Differential Diagnosis

- **Gout:** A crystalline arthropathy with periarticular/articular erosive changes centered around the metatarsophalangeal joints. Characteristic overhanging edges in the absence of osteopenia in an older male patient are most consistent with this diagnosis.
- *Rheumatoid arthritis:* An immune-based, symmetric, and deforming erosive arthropathy manifested by periarticular erosions with osteopenia typically seen in a female patient.
- *Septic arthritis:* A potentially destructive monoarticular process manifested by diffuse and gradual joint space loss with soft tissue swelling and eventual subchondral erosions.

■ Essential Facts

- Gouty arthritis is monosodium urate crystal deposition disease characterized by recurrent acute attacks of inflammatory arthritis.
- This disease is typically seen in 30- to 60-year-old male patients and is associated with obesity, hypertension, and regular alcohol consumption.

- Uric acid crystals are deposited in and around joints and may cause soft tissue fullness with or without amorphous mineralization, referred to as *tophaceous gout.*
- Typical gouty erosions are well marginated, sclerotic, and have a punched-out appearance with overhanging edges.
- Osteopenia is typically lacking.

■ Other Imaging Findings

- Dual-energy CT scanning may exhibit soft tissue tophaceous gouty crystalline deposits that are not readily evident on radiographs.
- Ultrasound findings may include joint effusions, synovitis, erosions, and echogenic uric acid crystals.

✓ Pearls and ✗ Pitfalls

- ✓ The initial attack of gouty arthritis is typically mono-articular, with erosions most commonly affecting the medial margin of the first MTP joint.
- ✗ Occasionally gouty arthritis may be superimposed upon osteoarthritis or rheumatoid arthritis, complicating the diagnosis.

Case 13

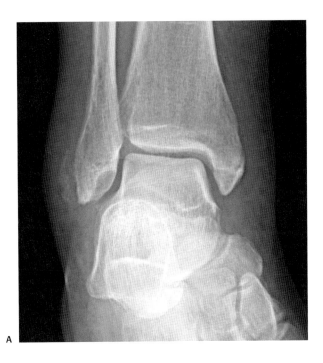

A

■ Clinical Presentation

A patient presents with a twisting injury to the ankle.

■ Further Work-up

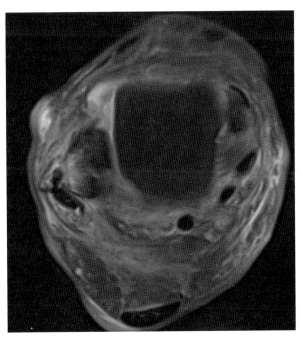

B

■ Imaging Findings

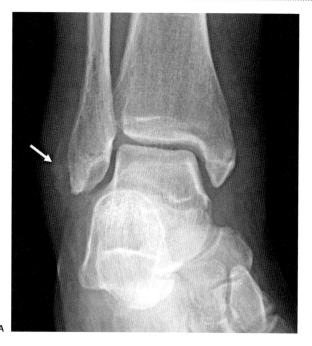 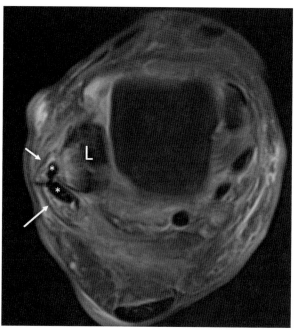

(A) Frontal radiograph of the ankle demonstrates a vertically oriented curvilinear avulsion (*arrow*) harvested from the lateral malleolus. (B) Axial fluid-sensitive MRI through the ankle at the level of the lateral malleolus (*L*) demonstrates lateral subluxation of the peroneal tendons (*asterisks*), which are positioned deep to the lateral malleolus bony avulsion (*short arrow*). The superior peroneal retinaculum (*long arrow*) adheres to this bony fragment.

■ Differential Diagnosis

- *Superior peroneal retinacular bony avulsion with lateral peroneal tendon subluxation:* A vertically oriented, longer than wide, bony avulsion positioned superficial to the lateral malleolus cortex resulting in lateral peroneal tendon subluxation along with elevation and detachment of the superior peroneal retinaculum are consistent with this diagnosis.
- *Supination external rotation–type fracture:* This injury accounts for the most common type of ankle fracture pattern, which is composed of a spiral lateral malleolus fracture, posterior malleolus fracture, and medial malleolus fracture.

■ Essential Facts

- Injury to the superior peroneal retinaculum results from forceful dorsiflexion of the tibial talar joint and frequently coexists with peroneal tendon dislocation.
- The peroneal tendons normally lie posterior to the lateral malleolus.
- One or both of the peroneal tendons may dislocate with this injury.

- A classification scheme exists for grading of superior peroneal retinacular injuries. A type I injury is the most common form, in which the superior peroneal retinaculum becomes detached from the lateral malleolus. A type IV injury involves a tear of the posterior portion of the superior peroneal retinaculum.
- MRI is the ideal imaging modality for evaluating these injuries, which may identify lateral and anterior peroneal tendon dislocation relative to the retromalleolar groove.

■ Other Imaging Findings

- Ultrasound may be utilized to elicit dynamic peroneal tendon subluxation and/or dislocation.

✓ Pearls and ✗ Pitfalls

- ✓ Lateral ligament complex injury frequently coexists with this type of injury.
- ✗ Depending on positioning of the ankle and the stage of injury, peroneal tendon dislocation may not be readily evident on MRI.

Case 14

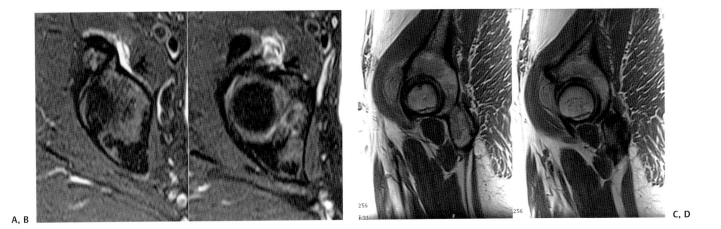

A, B

C, D

■ Clinical Presentation

A 42-year-old female presents with right groin pain and fullness.

■ Imaging Findings

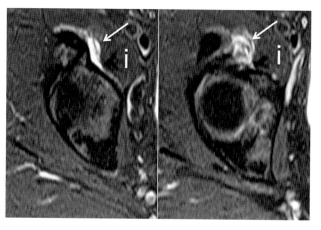
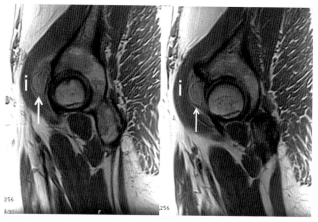

A, B

C, D

(A, B) Axial MRI fluid-sensitive images and **(C, D)** sagittal proton density fat-sensitive images through the right hip demonstrate heterogeneous fluid signal intensity (*arrow*) at the level of the iliopsoas (*i*) myotendinous junction.

■ Differential Diagnosis

- ***Iliopsoas bursitis:*** Posttraumatic versus inflammatory fluid/synovial distention of the iliopsoas bursa along the anterior margin of the right hip adjacent to the iliopsoas myotendinous junction represents this diagnosis.
- *Paralabral cyst:* A cystic hyperintense T2 focus on MRI which abuts the labrum and is contiguous with a labral tear are features of this diagnosis.
- *Iliopsoas tendon rupture:* Muscle and/or tendon fiber disruption with superimposed edema are consistent with this diagnosis.

■ Essential Facts

- The iliopsoas muscle is the primary hip flexor, composed of the psoas major, the psoas minor, and the iliacus muscle, which inserts upon the lesser trochanter.
- The iliopsoas bursa is the largest bursa in the human body and represents a synovial lined sac which serves as a protective buffer between the overlying musculature, tendons, and bony architecture of the hip.
- This bursa extends from the lesser trochanter to the iliac fossa, lying deep to the iliopsoas tendon and anterior to the hip joint.
- Fluid distention of the iliopsoas bursa may be seen with trauma, overuse, osteoarthritis, or inflammatory arthropathies.
- Mechanical aggravation of the bursa and tendon manifests clinically as internal snapping of the hip, with the iliopsoas tendon catching on a prominent iliopectineal eminence.
- MR findings may include increased soft tissue T2 signal with synovial thickening and/or bursal fluid distention along the course of the iliopsoas bursa and distal tendon.

■ Other Imaging Findings

- Real-time ultrasound imaging may display echogenic soft tissue and hypoechoic fluid at the level of the iliopsoas bursa, with potential iliopsoas tendon snapping upon provocative maneuvers.

✓ Pearls and ✗ Pitfalls

- ✓ An inguinal mass composed of mixed fluid and soft tissue density which extends along the course of the iliopsoas muscle into the lower pelvis/iliacus muscula-ture likely relates to iliopsoas bursal pathology.
- ✗ Inadvertent iliopsoas bursal contrast injection may occur during hip arthrography, manifested by contrast coursing in an oblique medial caudal to cranial fashion superimposed over the femoral head.

Case 15

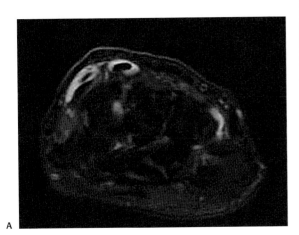

A

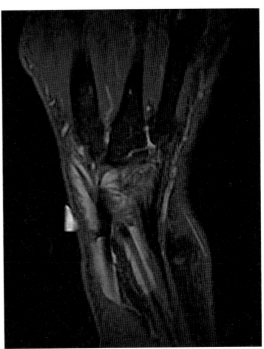

B

■ Clinical Presentation

A patient presents with dorsal wrist pain and swelling.

■ **Imaging Findings**

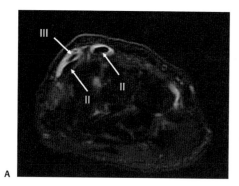

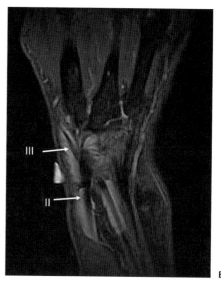

(A, B) Axial and coronal fluid-sensitive, fat-saturated MR images show isolated fluid signal intensity distending the tendon sheaths of the second (*II*) and third (*III*) extensor tendon compartments.

■ **Differential Diagnosis**

- ***Distal intersection syndrome:*** A focal inflammatory condition located at the intersections of the extensor carpi radialis longus/extensor carpi radialis brevis tendons (second extensor compartment) and the extensor pollicis longus tendon (third extensor compartment).
- *de Quervain's tenosynovitis:* Focal tendinopathy and stenosing tenosynovitis involving the first extensor tendon compartment.
- *Intersection syndrome:* Frictional tenosynovitis seen ~4 cm proximal to the distal radius secondary to the crossover of the abductor pollicis longus and extensor pollicis brevis tendons (first extensor compartment) and second extensor tendon compartment.

■ **Essential Facts**

- Distal intersection syndrome represents a noninfectious tenosynovitis at the intersection of the second and third extensor tendon compartments which occurs distal to the radiocarpal joint.
- Lister's tubercle is believed to be a factor in this syndrome, acting as a pulley and source of traction to irritate the extensor pollicis longus tendon.

- MR imaging may reveal interstitial tearing of the involved tendons along with fluid and synovial thickening.
- Severe cases may give rise to bone marrow edema within Lister's tubercle.
- Occasionally, this syndrome may follow a traumatic event.

■ **Other Imaging Findings**

- Ultrasound imaging may demonstrate hypoechoic tendon thickening with sonolucent peritendinous fluid at the intersection.

✓ **Pearls and ✗ Pitfalls**

- ✓ Severe cases of distal intersection syndrome may lead to periosteal reaction involving the underlying bony structures, potentially evident on radiographs.
- ✗ Distal intersection syndrome may coexist with intersection syndrome, complicating the diagnosis.

Case 16

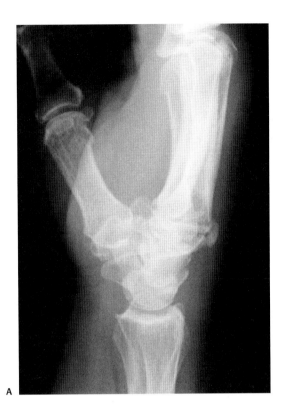

A

■ Clinical Presentation

A patient presents with a dorsal wrist mass.

■ Further Work-up

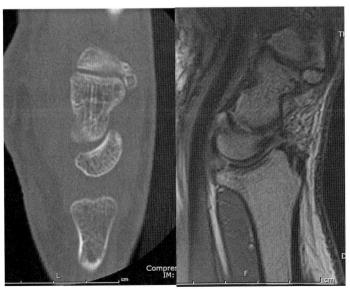

B   C

■ Imaging Findings

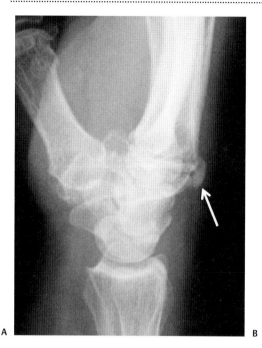
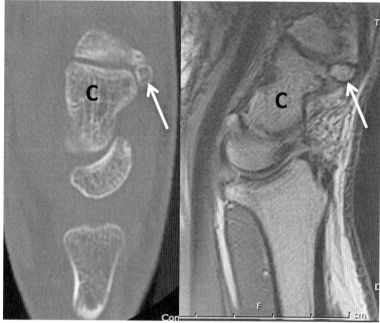

(A) Lateral radiograph of the wrist demonstrates a smooth corticated ossific density (*arrow*) positioned over the dorsal carpometacarpal (CMC) junction. **(B, C)** Sagittal CT and sagittal fat-sensitive MR images at the level of the capitate (*C*) demonstrate this ossific focus (*arrow*) intimately associated with the dorsal distal articular margin of the capitate (*C*) and the adjacent articular margin of the dorsal third metacarpal.

■ Differential Diagnosis

- ***Carpal boss:*** A dorsal bony prominence or ossicle positioned at the base of the second and third metacarpals and dorsal distal capitate.
- *Hydroxyapatite crystal deposition:* A basic calcium phosphate crystalline deposition disease typically seen within tendons and bursae around joints demonstrating decreased signal intensity on MRI and appearing calcified on radiography and CT.

■ Essential Facts

- *Carpal boss* refers to an underlying bony protuberance positioned between the bases of the second and third metacarpals and the dorsal distal capitate.
- This finding may be related to the presence of an osteophyte at this site versus an accessory ossification center referred to as an *os styloideum*.
- Patients may present with a palpable, firm dorsal wrist mass with or without pain and limited range of motion.
- MRI may reveal a ganglion cyst, bursa formation, or bone marrow edema in this region.

■ Other Imaging Findings

- Ultrasound imaging may reveal an echogenic focus continuous or separate from the adjacent metacarpal and capitate.

✓ Pearls and ✗ Pitfalls

- ✓ The carpal boss is best displayed on a lateral radiograph of the wrist utilizing 30 degrees of supination and ulnar deviation.
- ✗ Visualization of the carpal boss may be obscured secondary to the complex anatomy in this region.

Case 17

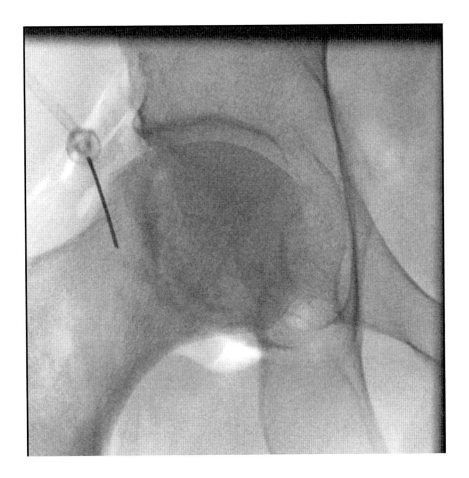

■ Clinical Presentation

A patient with chronic hip pain presents for a therapeutic steroid injection with an undocumented contrast allergy.

■ **Imaging Findings**

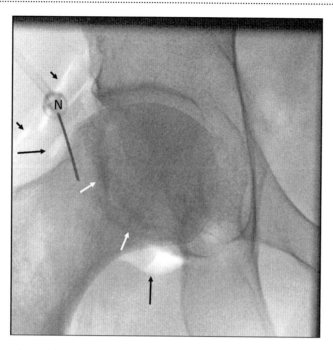

Fluoroscopic spot film of the right hip performed during a therapeutic steroid injection demonstrates a needle (*N*) along the superior femoral neck. A geographic rim of sclerosis (*white arrows*) encloses an area of heterogeneous sclerosis within the femoral head consistent with avascular necrosis. Hyperlucent intracapsular gas (*long black arrows*) conforms to the borders of the hip joint capsule. Linear hyperlucent streaks of gas (*short black arrows*) dissect within the surrounding tissues superior to the hip joint.

■ **Differential Diagnosis**

• ***Air arthrography:*** Insufflation of the hip joint capsule by injection of room air confirmed with hyperlucent gas conforming to the joint capsule on radiography/fluoroscopy.

■ **Essential Facts**

• Air arthrography may serve as a useful alternative to iodinated contrast administration in patients allergic to iodine.
• Room air is injected as a contrast agent.
• A well-formed hyperlucent intracapsular ring may be seen following injection of ~10 mL of room air into the hip.

• Major reactions to contrast injection may include anaphylaxis and vascular complications.
• Less severe complications associated specifically with intra-articular administration of iodinated contrast include chemical synovitis/pain, septic arthritis, and nerve palsy.

✓ **Pearls and ✗ Pitfalls**

✓ If a previous contrast allergy is known in advance, corticosteroids and antihistamines may be administered to counteract this reaction.
✗ Air arthrography performed prior to MR diminishes sensitivity and specificity of the exam secondary to susceptibility artifact and should be avoided.

Case 18

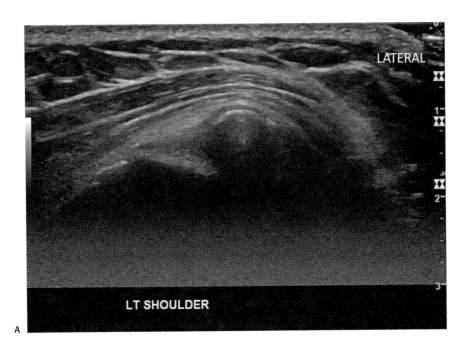

A

■ Clinical Presentation

A 50-year-old female presents with a several-months-long history of left shoulder pain with limited range of motion.

■ Further Work-up

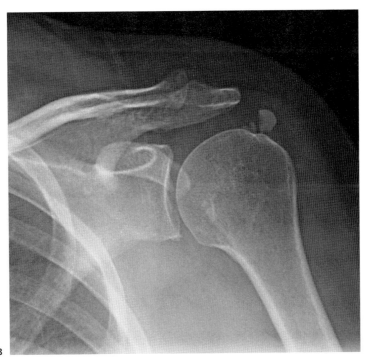

B

■ Imaging Findings

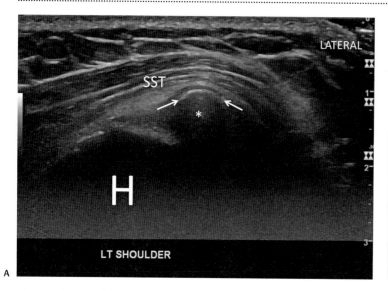
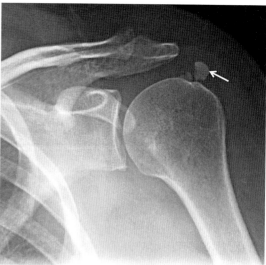

(A) Coronal-oriented ultrasound image through the left humeral head (*H*) demonstrates the supraspinatus tendon (*SST*). A curvilinear echogenic deposit (*arrows*) demonstrates posterior acoustic shadowing (*asterisk*) at the level of the supraspinatus tendon insertion onto the greater tuberosity. **(B)** Frontal radiograph of the left shoulder demonstrates calcific deposits (*arrow*) projecting adjacent to the greater tuberosity.

■ Differential Diagnosis

- **Hydroxyapatite deposition disease (HADD) of the rotator cuff:** Calcified and shadowing echogenic crystalline deposits positioned within the supraspinatus tendon in a 50-year-old female with pain and limited range of motion are consistent with this monoarticular degenerative crystalline deposition disorder.
- *Tophaceous gout:* Lobulated faintly calcified uric acid crystal deposits within a proteinaceous matrix associated with elevated uric acid levels are consistent with this diagnosis.
- *Calcium pyrophosphate deposition disease (CPPD):* Linear and diffuse calcifications which may be idiopathic or disease associated, sometimes indistinguishable from HADD.

■ Essential Facts

- HADD is a monoarticular disease process presenting between the fourth and seventh decades of life.
- Circumscribed calcific deposits may be associated with less intense symptoms than ill-defined amorphous deposits.
- This disease process is often referred to as *calcific tendinitis*.
- This process is characterized by calcifications in tendons near their osseous attachments.
- The development of these intratendinous calcifications is related to a combination of microtrauma and hypoxia as the calcifications are typically localized in poorly vascularized regions of tendons.

- Ultrasound imaging is ideally suited for this diagnosis given its ability to detect shadowing calcium deposits.
- This process is amenable to ultrasound-guided needling/fenestration, which enables partial or complete aspiration of deposits in addition to local bleeding to accelerate deposit resorption.

■ Other Imaging Findings

- MRI demonstrates intratendinous decreased T1 and T2 signal deposits with surrounding edematous inflammatory changes.

✓ Pearls and ✗ Pitfalls

- ✓ The most common site for these deposits is the shoulder, specifically the supraspinatus tendon.
- ✗ Partially resorbed hydroxyapatite crystals may exhibit decreased echogenicity with or without shadowing, making the sonographic diagnosis more challenging.
- ✗ Not infrequently, patients may present with a presumable infection.
- ✗ Collagen vascular diseases, along with multiple other metabolic disorders, may produce diffuse calcific deposits similar to hydroxyapatite crystals.

Case 19

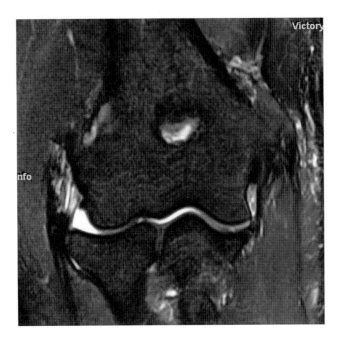

■ Clinical Presentation

A patient presents with chronic lateral elbow pain.

■ Imaging Findings

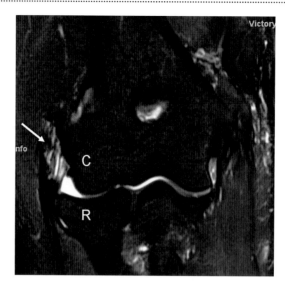

Coronal fat-sensitive MRI through the elbow at the level of the capitellum (*C*) and radial head (*R*) demonstrates hyperintense T2 signal (*arrow*) within the substance of the proximal common extensor tendon at the lateral epicondylar origin.

■ Differential Diagnosis

- ***Common extensor tendinopathy (tennis elbow):***
  A chronic degenerative tendinopathy of the elbow manifested by abnormal MRI signal increase related to interstitial tearing seen with overuse from excessive extension, supination, or gripping.
- *Common flexor tendinopathy (golfer's elbow):* Chronic degenerative tendinopathy of the elbow resulting from repetitive stress or overuse of the flexor pronator musculature. Patients present with a history of excessive forearm pronation and wrist flexion. MRI will display abnormal signal increase related to interstitial tearing.

■ Essential Facts

- Common extensor tendinopathy is also referred to as *tennis elbow* and *lateral epicondylitis.*
- Patients typically present with chronic and dull lateral elbow pain aggravated by wrist extension and gripping.
- The extensor carpi radialis brevis tendon is almost always the primary site of tendon pathology with variable involvement of the remaining wrist extensors.
- The extensor carpi radialis brevis tendon undersurface slides along the lateral edge of the capitellum during flexion and extension, potentially contributing to this tendinopathy.
- The deep fibers of the extensor carpi radialis tendon are poorly vascularized, which also potentially contributes to tendinopathy.
- MRI findings include interstitial tendon T2 signal increase, which relates to angiofibroblastic hyperplasia.

- Progressive interstitial tearing may eventually lead to full-thickness tendon disruption.
- This process may be amenable to ultrasound-guided tendon needling/fenestration, which enables local bleeding to accelerate healing.

■ Other Imaging Findings

- Ultrasound imaging demonstrates tendon enlargement and heterogeneity with areas of tearing depicted as hypoechoic regions of tendon fiber discontinuity. Echogenic shadowing calcifications may be seen within the tendon.

✓ Pearls and ✗ Pitfalls

- ✓ Common extensor tendinopathy is much more frequent than common flexor tendinopathy.
- ✓ Lateral epicondylar enthesophyte formation and/ or crystalline deposition may coexist with common extensor tendinopathy.
- ✗ Radiographs of the elbow are frequently noncontributory to the diagnosis.

Case 20

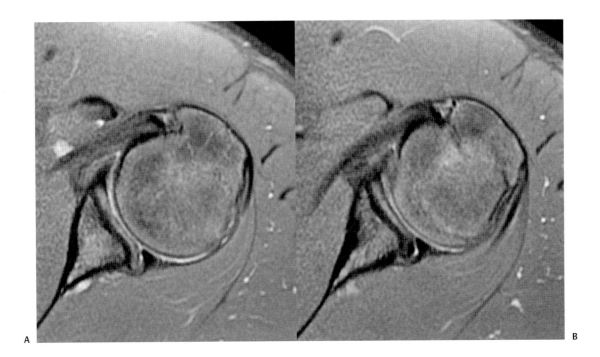

A

B

■ Clinical Presentation

A weightlifter presents with left posterior shoulder pain.

■ Imaging Findings

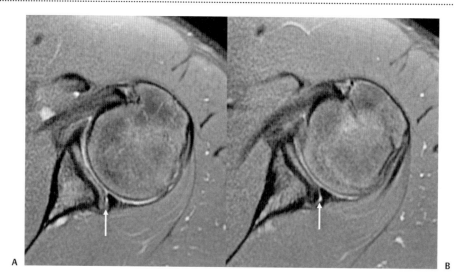

(A, B) Axial MR fat-sensitive sequences through the left shoulder demonstrate hyperintense T2 signal (*arrows*) extending through the base of the posterior labrum.

■ Differential Diagnosis

- ***Posterior labral tear:*** Axial MR imaging demonstrating hyperintense T2 signal disrupting the normal decreased signal of the posterior labral fibrocartilage is consistent with this diagnosis.
- *Sublabral foramen:* A normal variation of the anterior and superior labrum in which the labrum is separated from the glenoid margin.
- *Sublabral recess:* A normal cleft of varying depths normally seen on oblique coronal MR sections through the superior labrum. This recess is positioned between the glenoid hyaline cartilage and the base of the labrum and is oriented lateral to medial in a caudal to cranial direction.

■ Essential Facts

- Acute posterior labral tearing may be seen with posterior humeral head dislocations resulting from seizures, anterior shoulder trauma, and electrocution.
- Additional causes include repetitive microtrauma as seen with offensive linemen, baseball players, and bench pressing.
- MR arthrography demonstrates contrast extension through the posterior labral defect.

■ Other Imaging Findings

- Radiographs displaying ossification arising from the posterior and inferior glenoid into the joint capsule signify posterior labral pathology. This is referred to as a *Bennett lesion.*

✓ Pearls and ✗ Pitfalls

- ✓ Glenoid hypoplasia, also referred to as *posterior glenoid rim deficiency*, may coexist with posterior labral tearing.
- ✗ In the absence of significant acute trauma, standard non-MR arthrogram images may fail to display labral tears. Therefore, any history of dislocation or shoulder instability warrants MR arthrography.
- ✗ T2 signal increase related to joint fluid may insinuate between the joint capsule and the posterior inferior labral margin, mimicking a labral tear.

Case 21

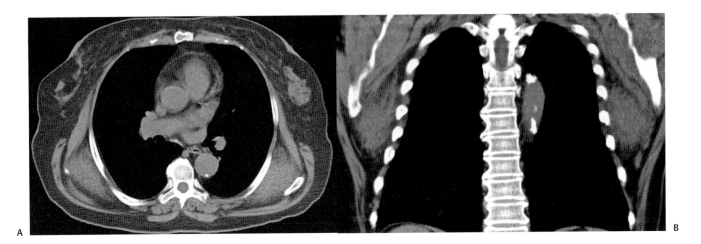

A

B

■ Clinical Presentation

An elderly female presents with a history of posterior chest wall masses.

■ Further Work-up

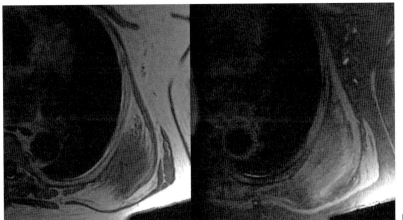

C

D

■ **Imaging Findings**

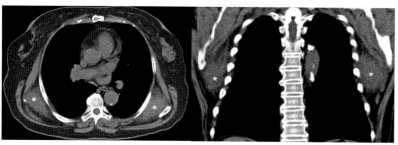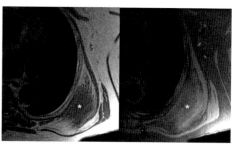

A, B   C, D

(A, B) Axial and coronal nonenhanced CT images through the chest demonstrate bilateral, symmetric soft tissue density masses (*asterisks*) containing irregular borders. These lesions are positioned inferior and deep to the distal margins of the scapulae. The masses are similar in density to the adjacent skeletal musculature. **(C, D)** Axial fat-sensitive and fluid-sensitive MR images through the left-sided mass (*asterisks*) demonstrate diminished T1 signal with T2 signal characteristics isointense to skeletal musculature.

■ **Differential Diagnosis**

- *Elastofibroma:* An infrascapular/subscapular solid, benign chest-wall mass seen in older patients demonstrating soft tissue density on CT scan and decreased T1/T2 signal on MRI.
- *Desmoid tumor:* A solid soft tissue fibrous/collagenous mass typically found in younger females of childbearing age seen in intra- and extra-abdominal locations.

■ **Essential Facts**

- Elastofibroma is a degenerative reactive fibrous pseudotumor arising from mechanical irritation adjacent to the scapulothoracic interface.
- These lesions may be seen in patients 55 years and older who present with stiffness and pain.
- The abundance of collagen deposition is responsible for the low-signal MR characteristics and CT attenuation similar to adjacent skeletal muscle.
- Bilaterality may be present in up to 60% of patients.

■ **Other Imaging Findings**

- Elastofibromas may demonstrate increased uptake on positron emission tomography scanning.

✓ **Pearls and ✗ Pitfalls**

✓ Elastofibromas have a right-sided predominance.
✗ These lesions are frequently overlooked when small in size, because they may be imperceptible from the adjacent skeletal musculature.

Case 22

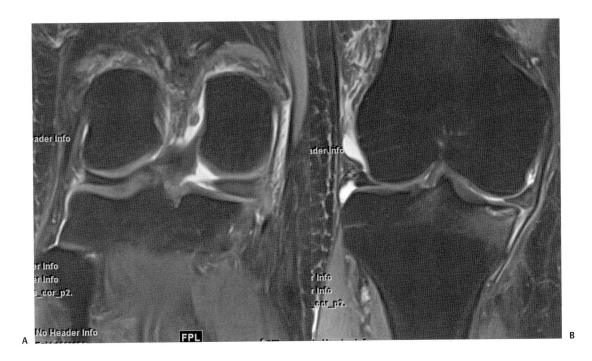

A

B

■ Clinical Presentation

A middle-aged female presents with a 1-month history of knee pain.

■ **Imaging Findings**

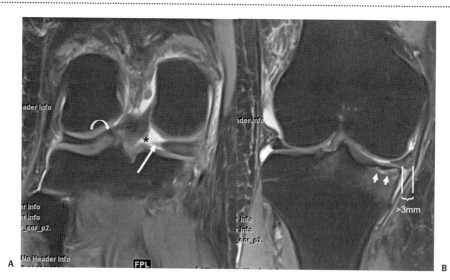

(A, B) Fluid-sensitive coronal MR images demonstrate fluid signal intensity (*asterisk*) extending through the posterior horn medial meniscus root insertion secondary to a radial defect. The disrupted irregular medial meniscus posterior horn root tissue (*long straight arrow*) is peripherally displaced. This results in > 3 mm peripheral extrusion of the medial meniscus body. Curvilinear signal alteration in the subchondral region of the medial tibial plateau with surrounding edema is seen (*paired short arrows*). The normal appearance of the posterior horn lateral meniscus root insertion (*curved arrow*) is used for reference.

■ **Differential Diagnosis**

• ***Medial meniscal root tear:*** A radial tear pattern occurring through the posterior horn of the medial meniscus root insertion resulting in peripheral extrusion of the medial meniscus body.
• *Bucket handle tear:* A displaced vertical/longitudinal tear typically seen in the medial meniscus resulting in a centrally displaced meniscal fragment which lies anterior to the posterior cruciate ligament (PCL), resulting in a "double PCL sign."

■ **Essential Facts**

• The meniscal root serves as the tibial attachment site for the meniscus, which assists with hoop stress displacement of forces traveling from the femur to the tibia upon axial loading.
• MR demonstration of hyperintense T2 signal disrupting the meniscal tissue in a plane perpendicular to the circumferential axis of the meniscus is consistent with a radial tear.
• This type of tear may disrupt the posterior horn medial meniscus root insertion and is ideally seen on coronal fluid-sensitive MR images.

• This results in abnormal axial loading from the femur to the tibia, causing high-grade medial compartment chondral loss.
• The development of underlying subchondral insufficiency fractures may occur, particularly in older female patients.
• Previously described as *spontaneous osteonecrosis of the knee* (SONK), the subchondral insufficiency fracture should prompt the radiologist to consider the possibility of an underlying medial meniscus root tear.

✓ **Pearls and ✗ Pitfalls**

✓ A posterior horn meniscal root tear should be suspected if meniscal tissue is not seen immediately adjacent to the tibial insertion of the PCL on sagittal MR images.
✓ Posterior horn lateral meniscus root tears have a high association with anterior cruciate ligament tears.
✗ The normal-appearing meniscal femoral ligament of the posterior horn lateral meniscus may cause confusion in diagnosing tears at the posterior horn lateral meniscus root insertion.

Case 23

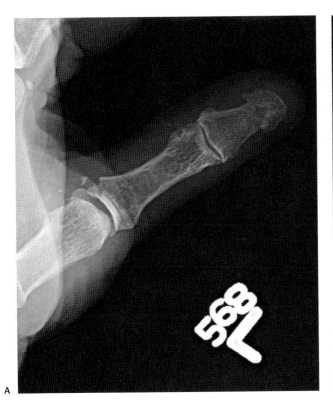

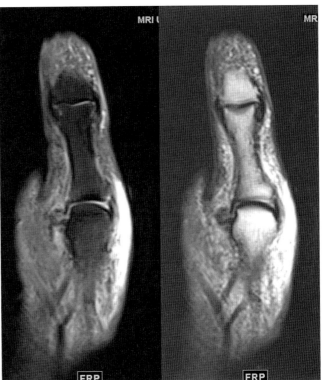

A

B, C

■ Clinical Presentation

A patient presents with a fall on an outstretched hand with the thumb abducted.

■ **Imaging Findings**

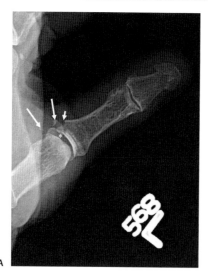 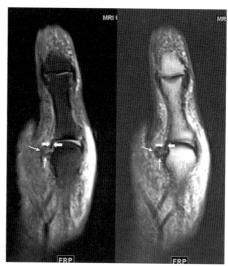

A   B, C

(A) Frontal radiograph of the thumb demonstrates a fracture defect (*short arrow*) at the ulnar corner of the proximal phalanx of the thumb. Displaced bony avulsive fragments (*long arrows*) are seen at the level of the medial thumb metacarpophalangeal (MCP) joint. Widening of the ulnar aspect of the thumb MCP joint (*asterisk*) is present. **(B, C)** Coronal fat-sensitive and proton density–weighted MR images through the dorsal aspect of the thumb metacarpal head demonstrate the adductor pollicis aponeurosis (*thick arrows*) positioned deep to a ruptured and proximally retracted, rounded and stumplike ulnar collateral ligament (*thin arrows*).

■ **Differential Diagnosis**

• ***Gamekeeper's thumb/Stener lesion:*** An avulsion fracture involving the medial base of the proximal phalanx of the thumb. Rupture of the ulnar collateral ligament allowing interposition of the adductor pollicis longus tendon deep to the ulnar collateral ligament is consistent with a Stener lesion.
• *Bennett fracture:* A fracture involving the articular base of the thumb metacarpal.

■ **Essential Facts**

• The gamekeeper's thumb derives its name from the valgus stress applied to gamekeepers when breaking the necks of rabbits.
• Also referred to as *skier's thumb.*
• Mechanisms of injury may include catching a ball or a fall on an outstretched hand with the thumb abducted.
• Radiographic findings of an avulsion fracture from the ulnar base of the thumb proximal phalanx may be seen in up to 40% of ulnar collateral ligament ruptures.
• Medial widening and/or radial subluxation of the thumb MCP joint are characteristic for this injury.
• The ulnar collateral ligament, which runs from the medial base of the thumb proximal phalanx to the medial thumb metacarpal head, may be ruptured.
• Tears of the ulnar collateral ligament are typically located distally at the thumb proximal phalangeal attachment.
• The adductor pollicis muscle and tendon, the primary dynamic stabilizer of the thumb MCP joint, is normally

positioned superficial to the ulnar collateral ligament and may be implicated in this injury.
• Additional forces following disruption of the ulnar collateral ligament allow the adductor pollicis aponeurosis to slide distal and/or deep to the ruptured ligament creating the Stener lesion. The malpositioning of these anatomic structures prevents normal healing.

■ **Other Imaging Findings**

• Ultrasound imaging may show a hypoechoic cleft through the ruptured ulnar collateral ligament.
• The ruptured and retracted ulnar collateral ligament manifests as a hypoechoic lobular mass on ultrasound imaging.

✓ **Pearls and** ✗ **Pitfalls**

✓ Markedly displaced avulsive fragments from the base of the medial thumb proximal phalanx typically coexist with a displaced ligament tear and/or Stener lesion.
✓ A nondisplaced avulsion fracture along the medial base of the thumb proximal phalanx does not necessarily exclude the presence of a Stener lesion or ulnar collateral ligament tear.
✗ Many gamekeeper injuries do not have associated fractures.

Case 24

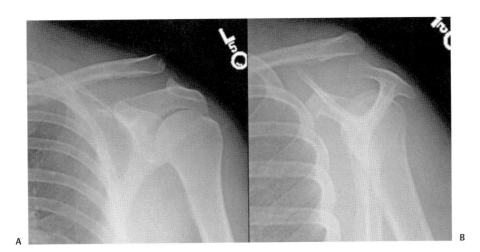

■ Clinical Presentation

A patient presents with trauma to the left shoulder.

■ Further Work-up

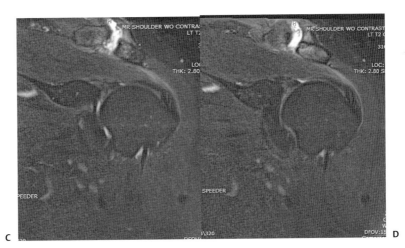

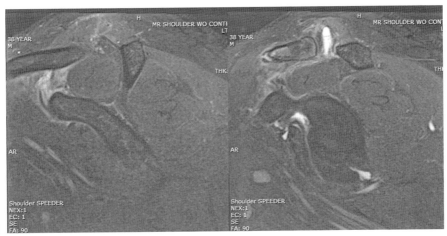

■ Imaging Findings

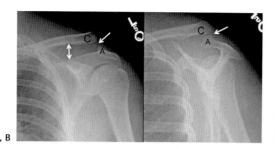
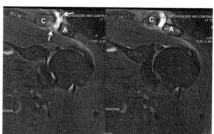

A, B

C, D

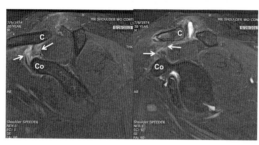

E, F

(A, B) Frontal and trans-scapular Y radiographs of the left shoulder demonstrate widening of the coracoclavicular interval (*double arrow*) with disruption of the acromioclavicular (AC) joint (*arrow*). There is elevation of the clavicle (C) relative to the acromion (A). **(C, D)** Coronal fluid-sensitive MR images through the shoulder demonstrate disruption of the superior and inferior AC ligaments (*arrows*) with fluid distention of the AC joint. Mild subcortical edema is seen within the distal articular margin of the clavicle (C) and acromion (A). **(E, F)** Sagittal fluid-sensitive sequences through the shoulder demonstrate signal increase with fiber interruption (*arrows*) through the coracoclavicular ligament between the distal clavicle (C) and coracoid process (Co).

■ Differential Diagnosis

- ***Grade 3 AC joint separation:*** A pattern of AC joint separation consisting of widening of the coracoclavicular interval, rupture of the coracoclavicular ligament, and 100% superior displacement of the clavicle at the AC joint.

■ Essential Facts

- Males are affected more commonly with AC joint injuries than females.
- AC joint injuries are commonly seen in rugby and American football.
- The Rockwood classification of AC joint injuries is the most accepted classification scheme.
- Rockwood grade 3 AC joint separation involves disruption of the AC and coracoclavicular ligaments with radiographs demonstrating > 5-mm widening of the AC joint and > 11-mm coracoclavicular interval widening.
- MRI findings of ligamentous disruption include disarray of ligamentous fibers with superimposed edema. Ligamentous sprains manifest with intrasubstance T2 signal increase without interruption of the fibers.
- Treatment of grade 3 injuries is controversial.

■ Other Imaging Findings

- Weightbearing radiographs may be used to discriminate grade 2 and 3 AC injuries demonstrating distraction of both the AC joint and coracoclavicular interval.

✓ Pearls and ✗ Pitfalls

- ✓ Disruption of the deltoid and trapezius musculature may be seen with grade 3 AC injuries.
- ✗ The superior margin of the AC joint may normally appear incongruent because the superior articular surface of the clavicle is positioned higher than the adjacent acromion.

Case 25

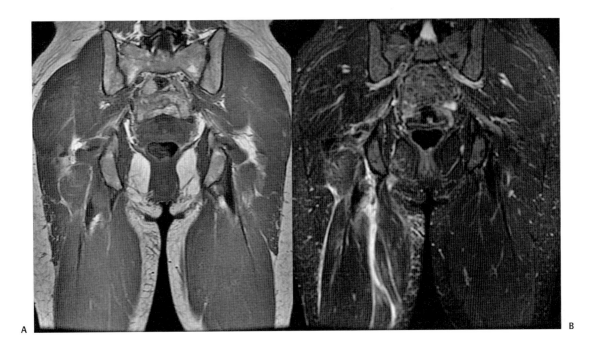

A

B

■ Clinical Presentation

A female triathlete presents with a fall from a bicycle.

■ **Imaging Findings**

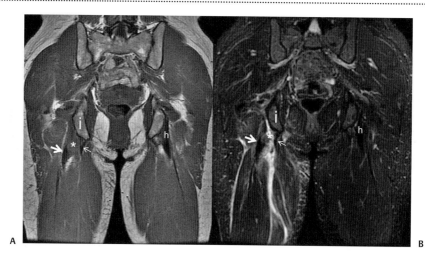

A   B

(A, B) Coronal fat-sensitive and fluid-sensitive MR imaging through the ischium (*i*) demonstrates focal tendon disruption with a fluid-filled gap (*asterisk*) at the origin of the right hamstring tendon complex. A distally retracted hamstring tendon (*thick arrow*) is demonstrated with surrounding muscle edema. The contralateral hamstring tendon complex (*h*) is intact. The right adductor magnus mini-hamstring tendon complex (*thin arrow*) is incidentally noted.

■ **Differential Diagnosis**

- ***Hamstring tendon rupture:*** A common athletic injury with MR imaging demonstrating fluid signal intensity replacing the proximal hamstring tendon at the level of the ischial origin with distal tendinous retraction and surrounding edema.

■ **Essential Facts**

- The hamstring muscles are important hip extensors and flexors.
- The hamstring tendon complex is composed of the biceps femoris, semitendinosus, and semimembranosus tendons.
- The biceps femoris and semitendinosus tendons are referred to as the *conjoined tendon* and originate from the posterior medial margin of the ischial tuberosity.
- The semimembranosus tendon originates in isolation from the superior and lateral margin of the ischium.
- Hamstring tendon injuries are typically seen in athletic activities that require rapid acceleration.
- Proximal hamstring tendon complex avulsion is the most serious acute injury of the hamstrings typically seen in adults.
- Hamstring tendon avulsions most commonly involve the entire proximal tendon complex. However, the conjoined tendon or, less frequently, the semimembranosus tendon may be ruptured in isolation.

■ **Other Imaging Findings**

- Ultrasound imaging may display diffuse focal tendon thickening and hypoechogenicity representative of tendinopathy, whereas tendon rupture manifests as hypoechoic fluid extending through the tendon defect.

✓ **Pearls and ✗ Pitfalls**

✓ Hamstring tendon avulsion in the adult skeleton typically occurs without an osseous avulsion, whereas the similar injury in the adolescent skeleton may result in an ischial apophyseal avulsive injury.

✗ The adductor magnus mini-hamstring tendon complex arises from the medial ischium and may be mistaken for a partially intact hamstring tendon slip.

Case 26

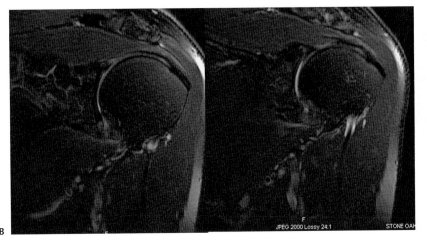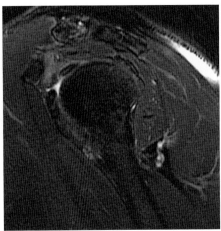

A, B   C

■ Clinical Presentation

A middle-aged female presents with restricted range of motion.

■ Imaging Findings

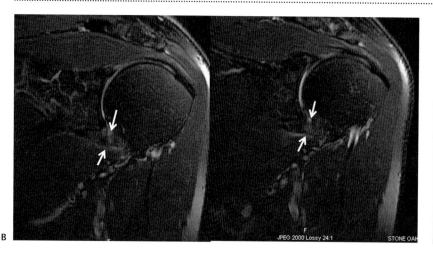
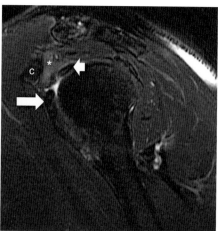

A, B

C

(A, B) Coronal fluid-sensitive MR images through the glenohumeral joint demonstrate an abnormally thickened and edematous joint capsule (*arrows*). **(C)** Sagittal fat-sensitive image through the rotator interval and coracoid process (*C*) shows signal increase/edema (*asterisk*) obliterating the subcoracoid fat. The subscapularis tendon (*long arrow*) and biceps tendon (*short arrow*) are seen.

■ Differential Diagnosis

- ***Adhesive capsulitis:*** An inflammatory condition frequently seen in middle-aged females with MR findings consisting of obliteration of the subcoracoid fat triangle with thickening and edema involving the inferior joint capsule.
- *Capsular sprain:* A posttraumatic stretch injury affecting the joint capsule, with MR findings of diffuse capsular edema with or without a joint effusion.

■ Essential Facts

- Adhesive capsulitis is an inflammatory condition of the shoulder joint capsule causing capsular thickening and contraction with limited range of motion.
- This condition is also referred to as *frozen shoulder.*
- This is a relatively common clinically diagnosed condition in the middle-aged female who presents with restricted range of motion which is worse at night.
- Adhesive capsulitis has been associated with conditions such as Dupuytren's disease, hyper- and hypothyroidism, and cerebral/cardiac and respiratory conditions.
- MRI findings include > 4-mm thickening of the coracohumeral (CH) ligament, capsular and glenohumeral thickening > 4 mm with obliteration of the subcoracoid fat signal intensity by edema.
- Adhesive capsulitis is considered a self-limited process.

■ Other Imaging Findings

- Shoulder arthrography may demonstrate diminished joint volume of < 10 mL with pain during and following injection.

✓ Pearls and ✗ Pitfalls

- ✓ A halo of edema outlining the axillary recess may be seen on sagittal fat-sensitive MR imaging.
- ✗ An undiagnosed early inflammatory arthropathy may have similar MR findings.

Case 27

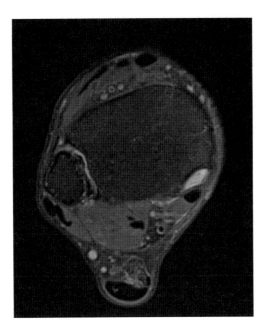

■ Clinical Presentation

A middle-aged female presents with flatfoot deformity and foot pain.

■ Imaging Findings

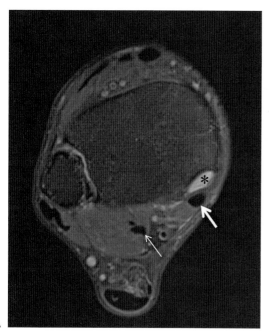
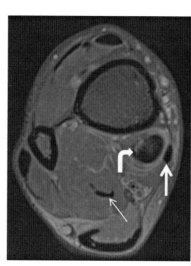
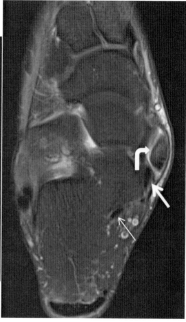

A   B, C

(A) Axial fat-sensitive MR imaging through the distal tibia and fibula demonstrates absence of the posterior tibialis tendon with a fluid-filled tendon sheath (*asterisk*) positioned medial to the flexor digitorum longus tendon (*thick arrow*) and flexor hallucis longus tendon (*thin arrow*). **(B, C)** Additional axial MR images proximal and distal to the medial malleolus reveal marked enlargement with signal increase within the posterior tibialis tendon (*curved arrow*).

■ Differential Diagnosis

• **Posterior tibialis tendon tear:** A common tendon derangement of the foot and ankle seen in the middle-aged female resulting in a flatfoot deformity. MR findings of an empty posterior tibialis tendon sheath at the level of the retromalleolar groove with retracted proximal and distal posterior tibialis tendon stumps are diagnostic features of a posterior tibial tendon rupture.

■ Essential Facts

• The posterior tibialis tendon assists with maintenance of the longitudinal arch of the foot.
• The posterior tibialis tendon primary insertion occurs along the medial navicular with smaller tendon insertions at the bases of the second through fourth metatarsals and the cuneiforms.
• Posterior tibial tendon tears are a chronic injury seen in females in the 5th and 6th decades presenting with a progressive flatfoot deformity.
• These tears are also common in obese patients and patients with inflammatory arthropathies.
• On axial imaging at the level of the medial malleolus, the posterior tibialis tendon should be no more than twice the size of the flexor digitorum tendon.
• Complete rupture of the posterior tibialis tendon is the least common type of tear and is termed a type III tear. More commonly, focal fusiform tendon enlargement with

interstitial tearing, or a type I tear, is seen. Focal tendon attrition and thinning, termed a type II tear, is second in frequency.

■ Other Imaging Findings

• Ultrasound imaging may demonstrate focal enlargement of the posterior tibialis tendon with linear hypoechogenicity representing type II tearing. Sonolucent fluid distention of the tendon sheath is seen with tenosynovitis. A type III tear of the posterior tibialis tendon will be manifested by an anechoic fluid-filled defect through the tendon.

✓ Pearls and ✗ Pitfalls

✓ Radiographs may reveal periostitis and/or a bony spur along the posterior medial malleolar groove related to the underlying tenosynovitis and tendinopathy.
✓ Spring ligament tears frequently coexist with posterior tibialis tendon tears.
✗ Non-weightbearing radiographs of the foot may not elicit midfoot collapse.
✗ MR signal increase within the posterior tibialis tendon adjacent to navicular insertion may normally be seen secondary to focal cartilage formation.

Case 28

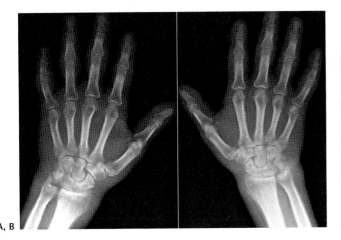

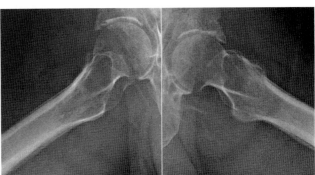

A, B

C, D

■ Clinical Presentation

A patient with polyarthralgias presents with weight loss and cough.

■ Imaging Findings

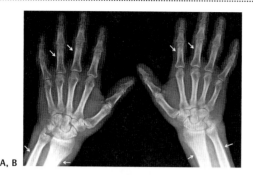
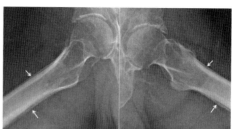
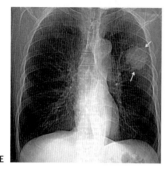

(A–D) Radiographs of the bilateral hands and hips demonstrate symmetric periosteal reaction (*arrows*) along the diaphyses of the phalanges, distal radii/ ulnae, and proximal femora. (E) Chest radiograph demonstrates a rounded opacity (*arrows*) in the left upper lobe consistent with bronchogenic carcinoma.

■ Differential Diagnosis

• ***Hypertrophic osteoarthropathy:*** Symmetric periosteal reaction of the tubular bones resulting from paraneoplastic syndrome related to bronchogenic carcinoma.
• *Rheumatoid arthritis:* A seropositive, autoimmune, symmetric, and deforming erosive inflammatory arthropathy.

■ Essential Facts

• Hypertrophic osteoarthropathy is a systemically mediated process demonstrating widespread periosteal reaction.
• Periostitis is usually accompanied by pain upon palpation to the involved area.
• Occasional clubbing of the fingers and toes may be seen along with soft tissue swelling.
• Effusions may be seen in larger joints.
• Primary and secondary forms of this condition exist.
• Bronchogenic carcinoma is one of the many secondary causes of diffuse periosteal reaction and occurs as a result of paraneoplastic syndrome.
• The bronchogenic carcinoma most frequently seen with this condition is adenocarcinoma, whereas small-cell carcinoma is the least frequently observed malignancy.

• Radiographs of the long bones demonstrate periosteal new bone formation.
• Patient symptoms and radiographic findings resolve following tumor resection.

■ Other Imaging Findings

• Nuclear medicine bone scan will show increased radio-tracer uptake at the sites of periosteal reaction.

✓ Pearls and ✗ Pitfalls

✓ Hypertrophic osteoarthropathy associated with lung cancer is typically symmetric, involving the diaphyses of the tubular bones with sparing of the epiphyses.
✗ An exhaustive differential diagnosis for secondary hypertrophic osteoarthropathy exists.

Case 29

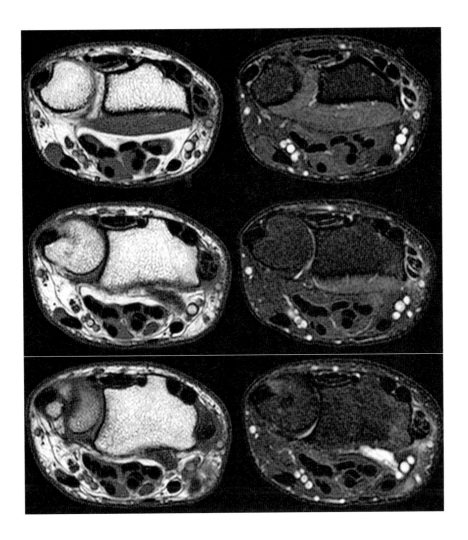

■ **Clinical Presentation**

A recreational tennis player presents with dorsolateral wrist pain.

■ Imaging Findings

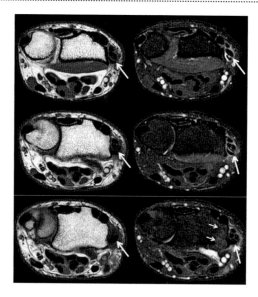

Axial fat-sensitive and fluid-sensitive MR images through the wrist demonstrate diffuse tendon enlargement with surrounding hyperintense T2 signal and fluid distention (*long arrows*) involving the first extensor compartment tendons. Focal subcortical bone marrow edema (*short arrows*) is seen within the underlying distal radius.

■ Differential Diagnosis

- ***de Quervain's tenosynovitis:*** Focal tendinopathy of the first extensor compartment tendons with surrounding soft tissue inflammatory changes and tenosynovitis related to overuse are consistent with this diagnosis.
- *Infectious tenosynovitis:* Focal tenosynovial thickening, with or without tenosynovial fluid associated with an underlying infectious process, is representative of this diagnosis.

■ Essential Facts

- The dorsal wrist is separated into six distinct extensor compartments.
- The first extensor tendon compartment is composed of the abductor pollicis longus (APL) and extensor pollicis brevis (EPB).
- de Quervain's disease is a stenosing tenosynovitis of the APL and EPB tendons in the first extensor compartment.
- Patients present with dorsal and lateral wrist/hand pain with limited range of motion of the thumb.
- This disease process is more commonly seen in females and is associated with repetitive gripping.
- Pregnant females are predisposed to this condition related to volume overload and hormonal effects.
- Nursing mothers may be affected secondary to mechanical stresses from supporting their infant's head.
- The disease may also be seen in athletes participating in racquet sports.
- Findings on MRI include thickening of the APL and EPB tendons with surrounding fluid in the tendon sheath.

■ Other Imaging Findings

- Ultrasound imaging demonstrates sonolucent fluid distention of the first extensor compartment tendon sheath with thickened hypoechoic tendons.

✓ Pearls and ✗ Pitfalls

- ✓ Wrist radiographs may demonstrate periosteal reaction along the radial styloid process secondary to the superimposed inflammatory changes.
- ✗ Variant anatomy of the APL tendon may mimic pathology.

Case 30

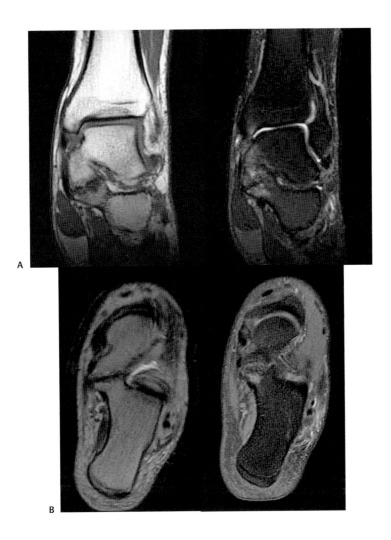

A

B

■ Clinical Presentation

A patient presents with chronic foot pain.

■ Imaging Findings

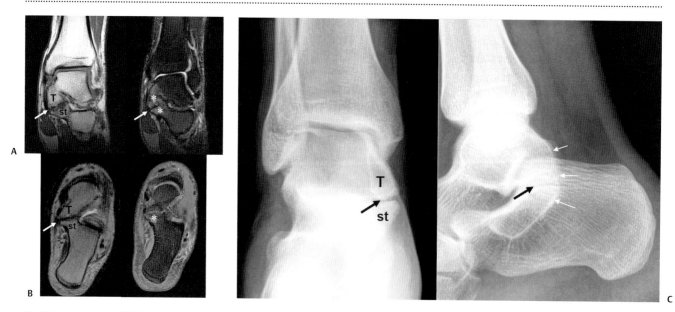

(A, B) Fat-sensitive and fluid-sensitive coronal and axial MR images through the middle facet of the subtalar joint (*arrow*) demonstrate subchondral bony irregularity along the articular surfaces of the talus (*T*) and sustentaculum talus (*st*). Superimposed bone marrow edema (*asterisks*) is seen at these sites. **(C)** Frontal and lateral radiographic projections of the ankle demonstrate a continuous "C" sign (*white arrows*) with narrowing and sclerosis across the middle facet of the subtalar joint (*black arrow*).

■ Differential Diagnosis

- **Talocalcaneal middle facet fibrous coalition:** A congenital segmentation abnormality involving the intertarsal joints. Middle facet subtalar joint articular irregularity with joint space narrowing, sclerosis, and bone marrow edema combined with a continuous "C" sign on lateral ankle radiographs is consistent with this diagnosis.

■ Essential Facts

- Tarsal coalitions are thought to originate from congenital osseous segmentation abnormalities.
- The most commonly affected bones are the talus, calcaneus, and navicular.
- Fusion occurs secondary to irregular fibrous, cartilaginous, or osseous tissue extending across an articulation.
- Talocalcaneal coalitions may coexist with a dorsal talar beak, as seen on lateral radiographs, related to traction from the calcaneonavicular ligament attachment and altered mobility of the subtalar joint.
- The continuous "C" sign may be displayed on lateral radiographs with a middle facet talocalcaneal coalition secondary to continuation of cortical shadows from the medial cortex of the talar dome and the cortex of the sustentaculum talus.
- Middle facet talocalcaneal coalition is the most common of the talocalcaneal coalitions.
- Patients typically present in adolescence complaining of stiffness, repetitive ankle sprains, and/or peroneal spastic flatfoot.

■ Other Imaging Findings

- CT scanning optimally displays osseous tarsal coalitions.

✓ Pearls and ✗ Pitfalls

- ✓ Tarsal coalition is bilateral in ~50% of cases.
- ✗ The "C" sign may be difficult to visualize on radiographic views if proper positioning is not achieved.
- ✗ Fibrous tarsal coalitions may be misdiagnosed as osteoarthrosis secondary to joint space narrowing with sclerosis.

Case 31

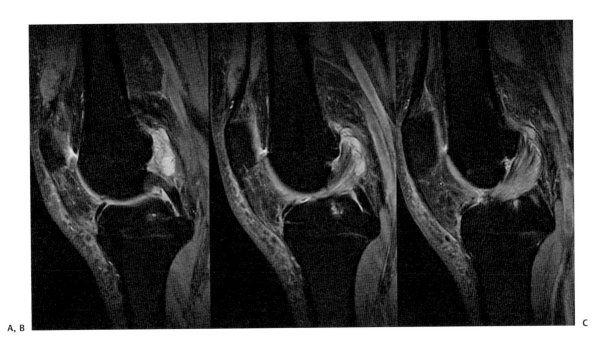

A, B
C

■ Clinical Presentation

A patient presents with chronic knee pain.

■ Imaging Findings

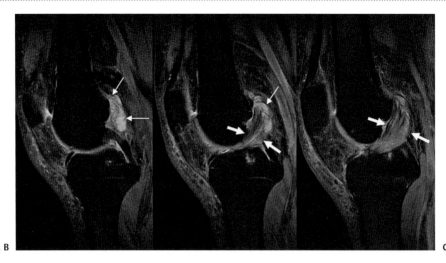

A, B   C

(A–C) Sagittal fluid-sensitive MR images display an intact anterior cruciate ligament (ACL) containing diffusely increased signal with a striated appearance (*thick arrows*) resembling a "celery stalk." An enlarged septated, heterogeneous hyperintense T2 cystic mass (*thin arrows*) is localized to the proximal ACL fibers.

■ Differential Diagnosis

• ***Anterior cruciate ligament mucoid degeneration with ganglion cyst formation:*** A degenerative process affecting the ACL resulting in an enlarged ACL containing linear increased MR signal intensity without discontinuity or rupture of fibers containing a mucoid cyst.

■ Essential Facts

• Both ACL mucoid degeneration and ACL ganglion cyst formation are thought to result from chronic mucinous degeneration of ACL connective tissue with or without antecedent trauma.
• These two entities are believed to represent a continuum of the same process.
• Incidence of these findings is reported at ∼1%.
• The celery stalk appearance derives its name from the interstitial mucinous degeneration causing a striated appearance on MRI as it expands the ACL tissue.
• Patients do not exhibit ligamentous instability.

■ Other Imaging Findings

• CT imaging through the affected ACL may demonstrate diffuse enlargement containing mixed soft tissue and fluid density with mucoid cysts demonstrating loculated fluid density.

✓ Pearls and ✗ Pitfalls

✓ Cystic intraosseous extension is typically seen along the bony margins of the affected ACL, possibly accounting for a patient's symptoms.
✗ Mucoid degeneration of the ACL may mimic an ACL partial tear/sprain on MRI.

Case 32

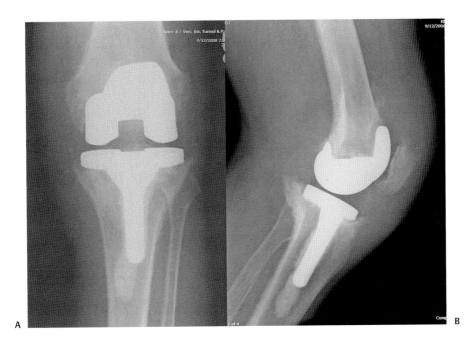

A   B

■ Clinical Presentation

A patient presents with a 2-week history of knee swelling and redness.

■ Imaging Findings

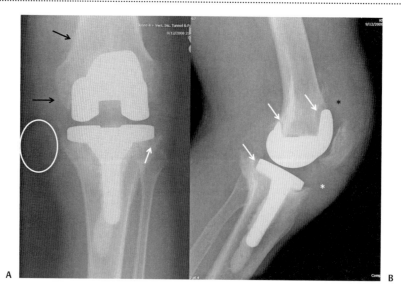

(A, B) Frontal and lateral knee radiographs demonstrate a knee joint effusion (*black asterisk*). Perihardware lucencies are seen about the femoral condylar and tibial implants (*white arrows*). There is marked infrapatellar soft tissue swelling (*white asterisk*). Periosteal reaction is seen along the distal femur (*black arrows*). Soft tissue gas (*encircled*) is seen over the medial joint line.

■ Differential Diagnosis

- **Hardware infection:** Osteomyelitis at the implant site of arthroplasty components with radiographic findings of soft tissue gas, swelling, joint effusion, and periprosthetic bone loss.
- *Particle disease:* A noninfectious, inflammatory process related to polyethylene particles shed from arthroplasty components. This process causes aggressive-appearing periprosthetic scalloped osteolysis on radiographs.

■ Essential Facts

- Hardware infection rate in patients after knee arthroplasty is < 2%.
- Infection in the acute phase tends to occur within 2 months of the operative date, whereas hardware infection in the intermediate phase may occur between 2 months and 2 years after surgery.
- The typical patient presentation is pain, not relieved by rest, with joint swelling and redness.
- Elevations of erythrocyte sedimentation rate and C-reactive protein are suggestive of infection.
- *Staphylococcus aureus* is the most common pathogen.
- Cardinal radiographic features include soft tissue gas, irregular osteolysis at the bone hardware interface, and soft tissue swelling.

■ Other Imaging Findings

- PET/CT with fluorodeoxyglucose (FDG) may be useful for detecting hardware and soft tissue infection exhibiting increased FDG uptake secondary to elevated glucose metabolism.

✓ Pearls and ✗ Pitfalls

✓ Periprosthetic lucency > 2 mm at the bone–hardware interface, or any new lucency around arthroplasty implants, should raise suspicion for loosening and possible infection.

✓ The presence of soft tissue or intra-articular gas in the setting of an infected joint is extremely specific.

✗ Radiographs are frequently normal in the setting of hardware infection.

Case 33

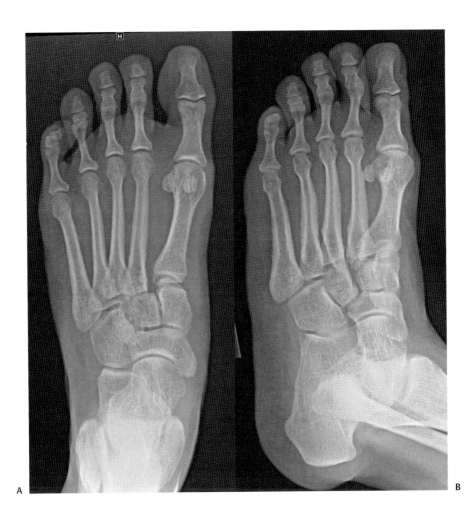

A

B

■ Clinical Presentation

A patient presents with a twisted foot with pain and swelling.

■ Imaging Findings

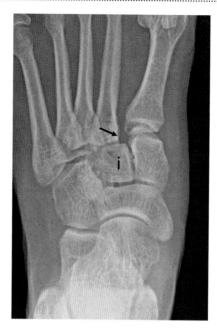

Frontal radiograph of the foot shows lateral subluxation of the second metatarsal base (*arrow*) relative to the intermediate cuneiform (*i*).

■ Differential Diagnosis

- ***Lisfranc ligament rupture:*** A traumatic ligamentous injury which may be associated with lateral second tarsometatarsal (TMT) joint subluxation.

■ Essential Facts

- Lisfranc ligament injuries and associated fractures result from abduction and/or plantar flexion to the forefoot causing distraction of the Lisfranc ligament.
- High-energy injuries such as motor vehicle accidents may lead to either a homolateral (first metatarsal base dislocates laterally) or divergent (first metatarsal base dislocates medially) dislocation across the TMT junction. The second through fourth metatarsal bases typically dislocate dorsally and laterally. Superimposed fractures through the bony articular margins are common.
- Low-energy injuries are more common in frequency and typically result in Lisfranc ligament sprains. The typical patient is a male athlete.
- Lisfranc ligament anchors the second metatarsal base to the medial cuneiform.
- On the frontal projection of foot radiographs, the medial cortex of the second metatarsal base should align with the medial cortex of the intermediate cuneiform. Malalignment at this site implies Lisfranc ligament disruption.
- Lisfranc ligament injuries must be surgically corrected to prevent the primary complication of degenerative osteoarthrosis.

■ Other Imaging Findings

- CT imaging may show subtle fractures along the course of Lisfranc ligament.
- MRI of Lisfranc ligament sprains will display intrasubstance signal increase, whereas ligamentous ruptures demonstrate absence of the normal ligament with superimposed T2 signal increase. Surrounding bony contusions are frequently seen in the adjacent osseous structures.

✓ Pearls and ✗ Pitfalls

- ✓ Foot radiographs may show disproportionate dorsal forefoot soft tissue swelling.
- ✗ Up to 20% of Lisfranc ligament injuries may present with negative radiographs.

Case 34

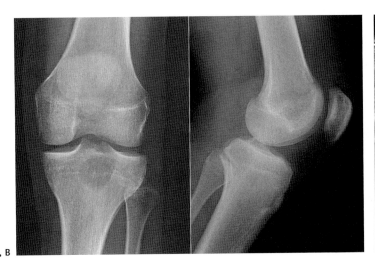
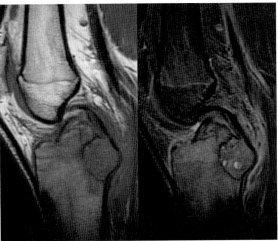

A, B   C, D

■ Clinical Presentation

An 18-year-old patient presents with knee pain and swelling.

■ Imaging Findings

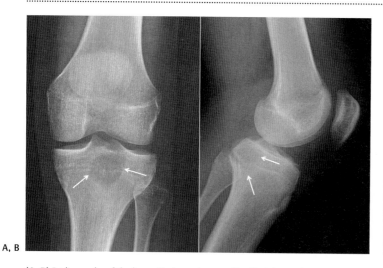
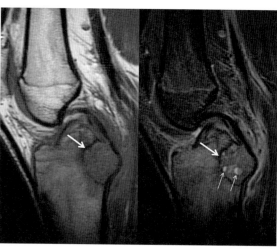

A, B   C, D

(A, B) Radiographs of the knee display a circumscribed lytic lesion (*arrows*) centered in the posterior aspect of the proximal tibial epiphysis. **(C, D)** Sagittal fat-sensitive and fluid-sensitive MR images through the lesion show intermediate to decreased heterogeneous T1 and T2 signal within the lesion (*thick arrows*) with surrounding marrow edema. Two small fluid–fluid levels (*thin arrows*) are seen on the fluid-sensitive MR image.

■ Differential Diagnosis

- **Chondroblastoma:** A benign epiphyseal-based cartilaginous lesion seen in the adolescent skeleton presenting as a circumscribed osteolytic epiphyseal lesion. MRI characteristics may include heterogeneous intermediate to decreased T2 signal with intense surrounding edema and fluid–fluid levels.
- *Brodie's abscess:* Typical imaging features of this infectious process include a lytic lesion on radiographs with MRI demonstration of a rim-enhancing intraosseous fluid collection.

■ Essential Facts

- Chondroblastoma is a benign cartilaginous neoplasm seen in the second and third decades of life.
- The typical patient presents with pain and swelling.
- Chondroblastomas arise in the epiphyses of long bones, most commonly the tibia, femur, and humerus.
- Radiographs demonstrate an epiphyseal-based circumscribed lucent lesion.
- Approximately 30 to 50% will have calcified chondroid matrix which may be detectable on radiographs and represented by signal voids on MR imaging.
- Malignant transformation is rare.
- Standard treatment is intralesional curettage.

■ Other Imaging Findings

- Nuclear medicine bone scan demonstrates increased radiotracer uptake on vascular and delayed phases.
- CT may demonstrate chondroid matrix calcifications which are not evident on radiographs.

✓ Pearls and ✗ Pitfalls

- ✓ Approximately 60% of these lesions will show low-intermediate T2 signal within the cartilage matrix with profound perilesional edema.
- ✗ Nearly 15% of chondroblastomas may show fluid–fluid levels on MR causing fusion with aneurysmal bone cysts.

Case 35

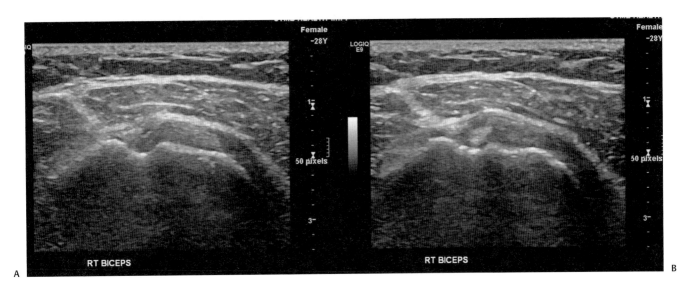

A

B

■ Clinical Presentation

A patient presents with right shoulder pain.

■ **Imaging Findings**

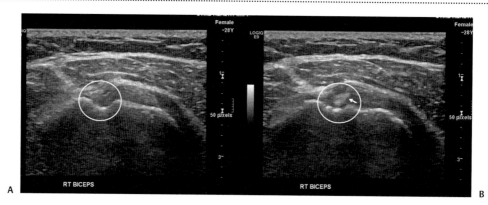

(A, B) Transverse sonographic images at the same level of the proximal right biceps sulcus (*circle*) demonstrate presence of the biceps tendon (*arrow*) on the right image with an empty biceps sulcus on the left image.

■ **Differential Diagnosis**

- ***Tendon anisotropy:*** An ultrasound artifact resulting in tendon hypoechogenicity or nonvisualization of the tendon related to inappropriate ultrasound beam angulation.
- *Biceps tendon rupture:* Sonolucent fluid replacement within an empty biceps sulcus secondary to tendon rupture and retraction.

■ **Essential Facts**

- Ultrasound evaluation of the shoulder is optimized by use of a linear array 12- to 15-MHz transducer.
- The ultrasound beam emission should be oriented perpendicular to the tendon fibers to maximize the reception of reflected sound waves from the tendon.
- An obliquely oriented transducer fails to receive all reflected echoes from the tendon, resulting in an artifactually hypoechoic or absent tendon.

✓ **Pearls and ✗ Pitfalls**

- ✓ This type of artifact may be eliminated by rocking the transducer along the respective axis of the tendon until the ultrasound beam has achieved the appropriate perpendicular angle.
- ✗ A large patient body habitus may require a curved 9-MHz transducer for appropriate penetration, increasing the occurrence of anisotropy.

Case 36

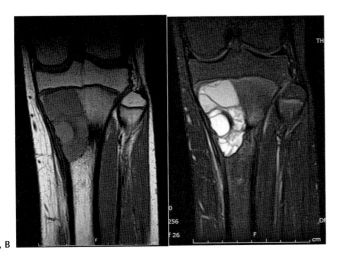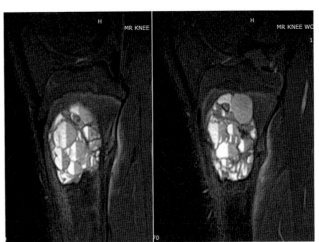

A, B   C, D

■ Clinical Presentation

A teenager presents with knee pain.

■ Imaging Findings

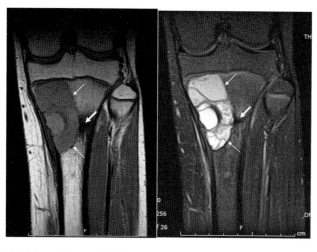 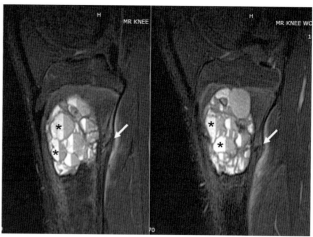

A, B   C, D

(A, B) Coronal fat- and fluid-sensitive MR images through the proximal tibia demonstrate a circumscribed, intramedullary lesion (*thin arrows*) within the proximal medial tibial metaphysis. Fluid–fluid levels (*asterisk*) are seen throughout the lesion on the sagittal fluid-sensitive MR images **(C, D)** A transversely oriented sclerotic region (*thick arrow*) with surrounding edema extends from the posterolateral margin of the lesion.

■ Differential Diagnosis

- **Aneurysmal bone cyst (ABC):** A localized lytic, expansile, benign bony lesion involving the metaphysis of a long bone exhibiting fluid–fluid levels on MRI is classic for ABC in this age group. A healing pathologic fracture abuts the posterior and lateral margin of this lesion.
- *Giant cell tumor:* A solid-appearing, circumscribed, heterogeneous, hypointense T1 and intermediate to hyperintense T2 lesion eccentrically positioned within the long bone epiphysis of an adult is representative of this lesion.
- *Simple bone cyst:* A uniformly hyperintense T2 cyst causing cortical thinning within a long bone in an immature skeleton is the typical MRI appearance for this lesion.

■ Essential Facts

- ABC represents a benign lesion of bone related to a reactive vascular process.
- Greater than 80% of primary ABCs occur in patients younger than age 20 years.
- These patients may present with localized pain and swelling.
- This lesion predominates in the metaphyseal region of long bones.
- Characteristic MRI features include a circumscribed intramedullary metaphyseal-based lesion with layering hemorrhagic fluid–fluid levels displayed on T2 imaging.
- Curative treatment is typically achieved with intralesional curettage.

■ Other Imaging Findings

- Radiographs typically show an expansile circumscribed lytic lesion in the metaphysis of long bones without internal mineralization or a soft tissue mass.
- CT imaging reveals expansion of the medullary canal with cortical thinning and no matrix mineralization.
- Nuclear medicine bone scanning may show a central photopenic region referred to as the "doughnut sign."

✓ Pearls and ✕ Pitfalls

- ✓ Spinal ABCs tend to involve the posterior elements.
- ✕ Several solid bony lesions may exhibit secondary aneurysmal bone cyst changes complicating the diagnosis.

Case 37

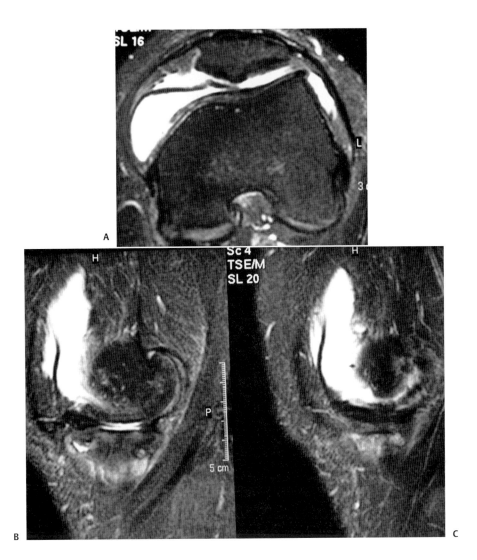

■ Clinical Presentation

A patient presents with chronic medial knee pain with clicking over the medial patellofemoral joint upon flexion and extension.

■ Imaging Findings

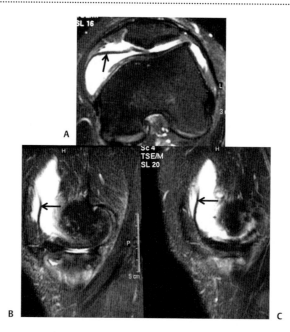

(A–C) Axial and sagittal fluid-sensitive MR sequences through the knee demonstrate a low signal intensity thickened bandlike structure (*arrow*) emanating from the medial wall of the knee joint, partially incarcerated between the patella and the femur. A large joint effusion is present with thinning of the patellofemoral cartilage.

■ Differential Diagnosis

• **Medial plica syndrome of the knee:** A symptomatic synovial septal remnant seen along the medial aspect of the patellofemoral joint. This structure appears as a thickened and linear low MR signal intensity band over the medial patellofemoral joint and may cause high-grade patellar and femoral chondral loss.

■ Essential Facts

• Synovial plicae are normal anatomic thin, pliable synovial folds.
• Plica syndrome refers to pain in the knee in which the primary finding explaining patients' symptoms is the presence of a thickened plica.
• The medial patellar plica is the most symptomatic.
• Patients present with medial joint pain typically just superior to the medial patellofemoral joint.
• The thickened medial plica may present as a palpable cord that causes clicking on flexion and extension of the patellofemoral joint.
• The thickened and fibrotic plica demonstrates low signal on MR imaging.
• Repetitive friction from grinding of the thickened plica between the chondral surfaces of the patellofemoral joint leads to progressive chondral loss.
• Treatment includes arthroscopic resection of the thickened plica.

■ Other Imaging Findings

• Ultrasound imaging may demonstrate real-time transient patellofemoral incarceration of the medial plica with flexion and extension maneuvers.

✓ Pearls and ✗ Pitfalls

✓ The diagnosis of plicae syndrome may be suggested in the presence of thickening of a single plica with adjacent chondral bony erosions and a joint effusion with the absence of other internal derangements.
✗ No consistent measurement exists regarding the normal thickness of a plica.

Case 38

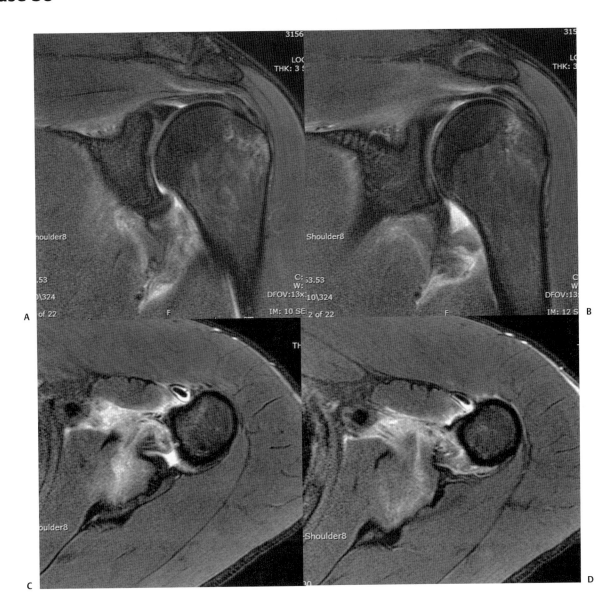

■ Clinical Presentation

A patient with a history of a fall from a ladder presents with shoulder pain.

■ Imaging Findings

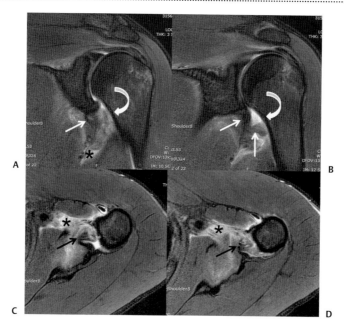

(A–D) Coronal and axial fluid-sensitive MR images through the shoulder joint show marked edema (*asterisks*) outlining the inferior glenohumeral joint capsule and adjacent axillary soft tissues. The inferior glenohumeral ligament (*white arrows*) is detached from the proximal humeral attachment (*curved arrows*) and appears thickened and edematous. The ruptured inferior glenohumeral ligament (*black arrows*) shows medial retraction.

■ Differential Diagnosis

• ***Humeral avulsion of the glenohumeral ligament (HAGL):***
A traumatic ligamentous avulsion injury seen at the level of the shoulder joint. MRI demonstrates thickening and edema of the inferior glenohumeral ligament with associated humeral detachment.

■ Essential Facts

• The inferior glenohumeral ligament is a hammocklike structure with anterior and posterior bands connected by the axillary recess.
• This ligament extends from the anterior inferior labral region to the surgical neck of the humerus.
• The HAGL lesion is typically seen with anterior shoulder dislocations.
• These injuries manifest on MRI with periarticular edema and hemorrhage localized to the axillary pouch, quadrilateral space, and proximal humerus.
• Humeral bony avulsions are seen with ~20% of these injuries.

■ Other Imaging Findings

• Arthrography may reveal inferior and medial contrast extravasation through the glenohumeral ligament defect.

✓ Pearls and ✗ Pitfalls

✓ Other injuries that may be seen in conjunction with the HAGL lesion include anterior-inferior labral tears, anterior-inferior glenoid articular cartilage defects, and/or bony glenoid defects.
✗ Inferior glenohumeral ligament injury may be overestimated in the setting of hemorrhage.

Case 39

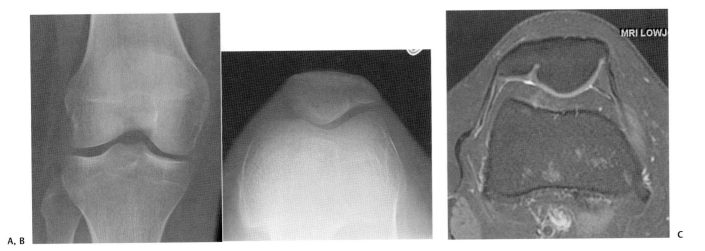

A, B

C

■ Clinical Presentation

A patient presents with an abnormality seen on knee radiographs.

■ Imaging Findings

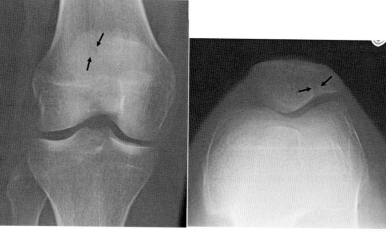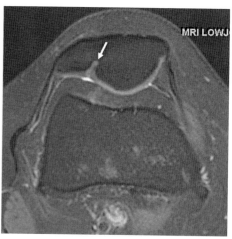

A, B

C

(A, B) Frontal and axial radiographs of the knee demonstrate a round lucent lesion (*arrows*) along the dorsal superior and lateral surface of the patellar articular surface. **(C)** Axial fluid-sensitive MR imaging through the knee demonstrates invagination of articular cartilage and the subchondral bone plate (*arrow*) at the level of the lateral patellar facet.

■ Differential Diagnosis

• **Dorsal defect of the patella (DDP):** A congenital circumscribed lucency through the lateral facet of the patella related to invagination of cartilage.
• *Osteochondral defect:* A posttraumatic partial or full-thickness articular cartilage surface defect with or without associated bone marrow edema.

■ Essential Facts

• DDP represents a patellar variant seen in 0.5 to 1% of the population.
• This defect is most commonly discovered incidentally and rarely presents with pain.
• This defect is localized to the lateral patellar facet and demonstrates invagination of the articular cartilage into the subchondral bone on MRI.
• Radiographs demonstrate a superolateral patellar articular-sided round lucency that is best outlined on axial patellar views.
• Disappearance of these defects may occur over time.

■ Other Imaging Findings

• CT scan will demonstrate a cortical defect outlined by sclerosis along the lateral patellar facet filled in with soft tissue density representing cartilage.

✓ Pearls and ✗ Pitfalls

✓ The cartilage overlying the DDP is typically intact, in contrast to an osteochondral injury.
✗ Suboptimal positioning of knee radiographs may limit detection of this variant.

Case 40

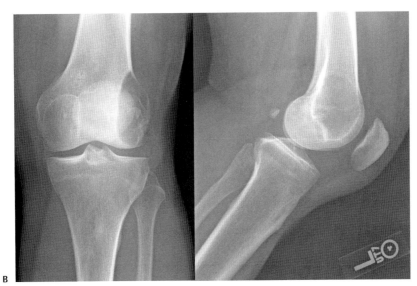

A, B

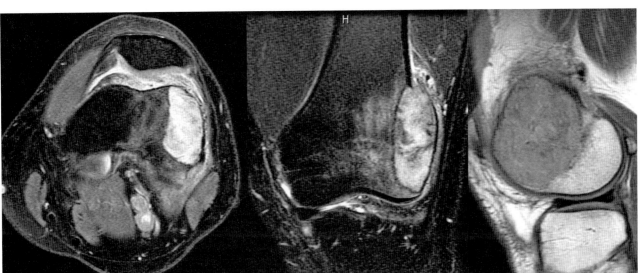

H

C

D, E

■ Clinical Presentation

A 40-year-old patient presents with knee pain.

■ Imaging Findings

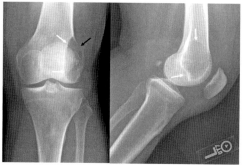
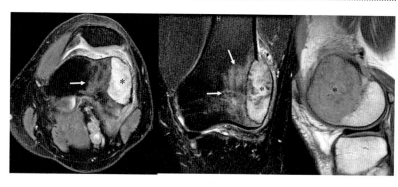

A, B   C, D,

(A, B) Frontal and lateral radiographs of the knee demonstrate an eccentric, expansile, geographic, lytic lesion (*white arrows*) centered in the meta-epiphysis of the lateral femoral condyle extending to the subchondral bone. This lesion causes marked thinning of the lateral cortex (*black arrow*). There is lack of internal mineralization. **(C–E)** Fluid-sensitive and fat-sensitive MR images show marrow replacement with mixed hypo- and hyperintense T1 and T2 signal within the lesion (*asterisks*) with surrounding perilesional edema (*white arrows*). No soft tissue mass is present.

■ Differential Diagnosis

- *Giant cell tumor (GCT):* A benign meta-epiphyseal–based lytic lesion seen in the adult skeleton associated with cortical thinning and mixed T1/T2 MR signal.
- *Chondroblastoma:* A benign epiphyseal-based cartilaginous lesion seen in the adolescent skeleton.
- *Intraosseous ganglion:* A subcortical, intraosseous simple cystlike structure likely degenerative in etiology.

■ Essential Facts

- GCT accounts for ~20% of benign bone neoplasms.
- These lesions are typically solitary.
- Patients can present with pain, local swelling, or pathologic fractures.
- The most common location of GCT is about the knee.
- GCT may develop in the skull, pelvis, or facial bones in patients with Paget's disease.
- The circumscribed radiographic lytic changes seen with this tumor relate to bone destruction by osteoclastic giant cells which are diffusely distributed throughout the tumor.
- The MRI features consist of a circumscribed intramedullary lesion containing decreased T1 and heterogeneous increased T2 signal.
- Blood products with hemosiderin may be seen within the lesion demonstrating diminished T1 and T2 signal on MRI.
- Secondary aneurysmal bone cyst formation may occur with MRI demonstrating fluid–fluid levels.
- Traditional treatment consists of curettage and cement packing.
- Recurrence may be seen in up to 25% of cases.

■ Other Imaging Findings

- CT scan shows lack of mineralization within the lesion with thinning of the cortices.
- Nuclear medicine bone scan typically shows increased radiotracer uptake along the perimeter of the lesion with central photopenia related to osteolysis and/or necrosis.

✓ Pearls and ✗ Pitfalls

- ✓ These lesions extend to within 1 cm of the subarticular bone and typically occur in patients with closed physes.
- ✗ GCTs may occasionally have aggressive features including a wide zone of transition with cortical thinning, bone destruction, and an associated soft tissue mass.

Case 41

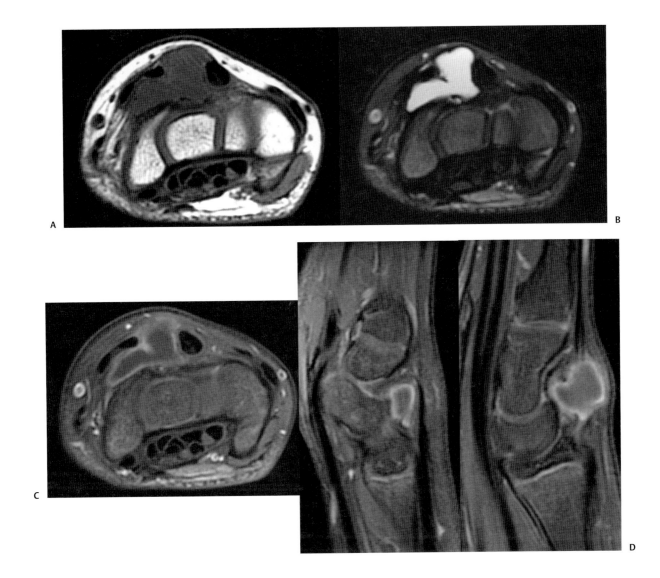

■ Clinical Presentation

A patient presents with a dorsal wrist mass.

■ **Imaging Findings**

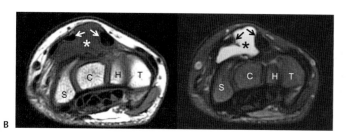 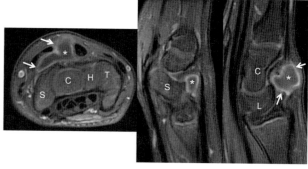

A, B   C, D

(A, B) Axial fat-sensitive and fluid-sensitive MR images through the proximal wrist at the level of the scaphoid (*S*), capitate (*C*), hamate (*H*), and triquetrum (*T*) demonstrate a cystic mass (*asterisk*) displacing the overlying extensor tendons (*arrows*). **(C, D)** Axial and sagittal fat-suppressed post-gadolinium images at the level of the lunate (*L*), capitate (*C*), and scaphoid (*S*) demonstrate rim enhancement (*white arrows*) surrounding the soft tissue mass (*asterisks*).

■ **Differential Diagnosis**

- *Ganglion cyst:* A degenerative juxta-articular soft tissue mass with MR fluid signal characteristics demonstrating rim enhancement after gadolinium administration.
- *Vascular malformation:* An acquired vascular lesion with arterial/venous shunting exhibiting solid and/or variable contrast enhancement.
- *Synovial sarcoma:* A solid malignant lesion with aggressive growth characteristics with variable MRI signal characteristics exhibiting heterogeneous enhancement with or without calcifications.

■ **Essential Facts**

- Ganglion cysts represent encapsulated myxomatous degenerative tissue located adjacent to joints, ligaments, or tendons.
- The origin of ganglion cysts is not uniformly agreed upon. However, a traumatic etiology is likely.
- Dorsal carpal ganglion cysts are most common and occur over the scapholunate ligament which may or may not be injured.
- Ganglion cysts should not be confused with synovial cysts, which are lined by synovium and contain synovial fluid.
- The ganglion cyst is lined by fibrous tissue which will enhance following IV gadolinium administration.
- The internal myxomatous contents of the cyst exhibits homogeneous hypointense T1 and hyperintense T2 signal. Internal septations may occur with larger cysts.
- Careful inspection of radiographs may reveal a protuberant and rounded soft tissue density.
- Surgical resection is commonly required for prevention of recurrence.

■ **Other Imaging Findings**

- Ultrasound imaging demonstrates a circumscribed anechoic cystic mass with posterior acoustic enhancement.

✓ **Pearls and ✗ Pitfalls**

✓ The most common palpable soft tissue mass around the wrist is a ganglion cyst.
✓ Ganglion cysts do not calcify.
✗ Not all ganglion cysts are simple in appearance and may be hemorrhagic, septated, or partially ruptured, complicating the diagnosis on MRI and ultrasound.

Case 42

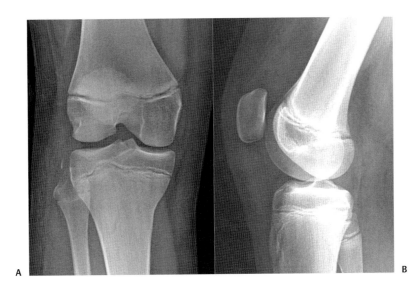

A   B

■ Clinical Presentation

A patient presents with a knee sprain and lateral joint line tenderness with instability.

■ Further Work-up

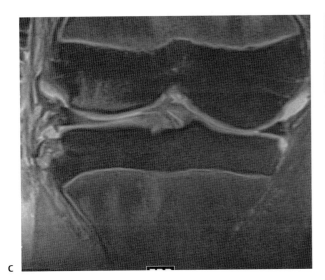

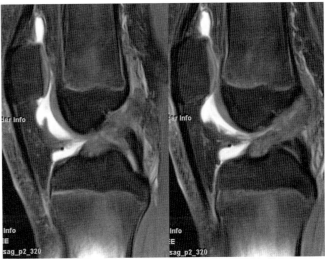

C   D, E

■ Imaging Findings

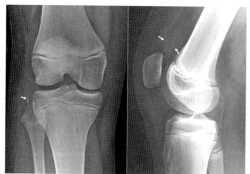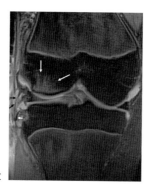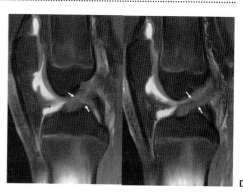

A, B   C   D, E

(A, B) Radiographs of the knee demonstrate a linear avulsion fracture (*arrow*) adjacent to the lateral plateau. A joint effusion is present (*arrows*).
(C) Coronal fluid-sensitive MR image shows a bone contusion within the lateral femoral condyle (*long white arrows*). A curvilinear low-signal cortical avulsion (*short white arrow*) adheres to a thin ligamentous structure (*short black arrows*) that also attaches to the periphery of the lateral meniscus.
(D, E) Sagittal fluid-sensitive MR images show a torn anterior cruciate ligament (ACL; *arrows*).

■ Differential Diagnosis

- **Segond fracture:** A middle third lateral tibial capsular ligamentous avulsion fracture resulting from a twisting injury with a high association with ACL tears.
- *Arcuate sign:* This fracture is associated with a high-energy hyperextension injury resulting in a bony avulsion from the fibular head at the attachment of the arcuate ligament. Cruciate and posterior lateral corner ligament injuries may also be seen.

■ Essential Facts

- Segond fracture represents an avulsion injury from the proximal tibia just distal to the lateral tibial plateau.
- This injury is caused by forceful internal rotation and varus stress.
- Patients present with lateral joint line pain and rotational instability.
- This fragment is typically harvested from the middle third lateral capsular ligament tibial insertion posterior to Gerdy's tubercle of the tibia.
- This avulsive fragment is best displayed on frontal knee radiographs adjacent to the lateral tibial plateau.
- There is a 75 to 100% association with ACL tears, which are readily diagnosable on MRI.
- Radiographic findings of vertically oriented bony remodeling or a longitudinal bony excrescence just below the lateral tibial plateau should raise suspicion for a chronic Segond avulsion and ACL incompetency.

■ Other Imaging Findings

- Radionuclide bone scan will show increased radiotracer uptake at the fracture sites.

✓ Pearls and ✗ Pitfalls

- ✓ The morphology of the Segond avulsive fragment is typically elliptical and parallel to the tibial longitudinal axis.
- ✗ The fragment may be thinned and/or nondisplaced, limiting detection on radiographs.

Case 43

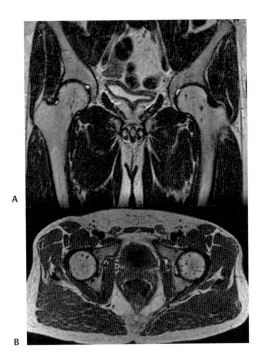

A

B

■ Clinical Presentation

A male patient presents with hip pain.

■ Imaging Findings

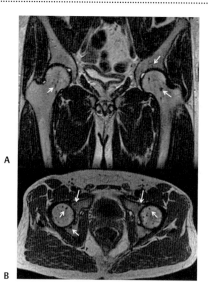

(**A, B**) Coronal T2 and axial T1 MR images of the pelvis demonstrate innumerable, symmetric, low-signal ovoid lesions (*arrows*) surrounding both hip joints.

■ Differential Diagnosis

- ***Osteopoikilosis:*** A bone-forming dystrophy resulting in symmetric bone islands in a periarticular distribution.
- *Metastasis:* Blastic bony lesions resulting from a primary malignancy causing asymmetric, variable-sized sclerotic lesions involving the axial and appendicular skeleton.
- *Mastocytosis:* A mast cell proliferative disorder exhibiting asymmetric and less well-defined sclerotic lesions without a periarticular predominance.

■ Essential Facts

- Osteopoikilosis falls into a category of benign diseases referred to as the *bone-forming dystrophies.*
- This is an asymptomatic process which may be evident at any age and tends to be symmetric.
- These sclerotic and spiculated lesions are typically < 1 cm and may enlarge, stabilize, or disappear over time.
- There is a predilection for these skeletal changes to occur in the meta-epiphyseal regions of long/tubular bones, pelvis, scapula, and carpus/tarsus.
- The bony changes are related to islands of compact bone.
- MRI findings include low T1/T2 subcentimeter spiculated bony lesions in a periarticular distribution.

■ Other Imaging Findings

- Radiography and CT imaging reveal multiple ovoid, symmetric, and sclerotic densities.

✓ Pearls and ✗ Pitfalls

- ✓ Osteopoikilosis is rare in the spine and skull and typically does not show increased uptake on nuclear medicine bone scan.
- ✗ Overlapping syndromes with other sclerosing bone-forming dystrophies may occur.

Case 44

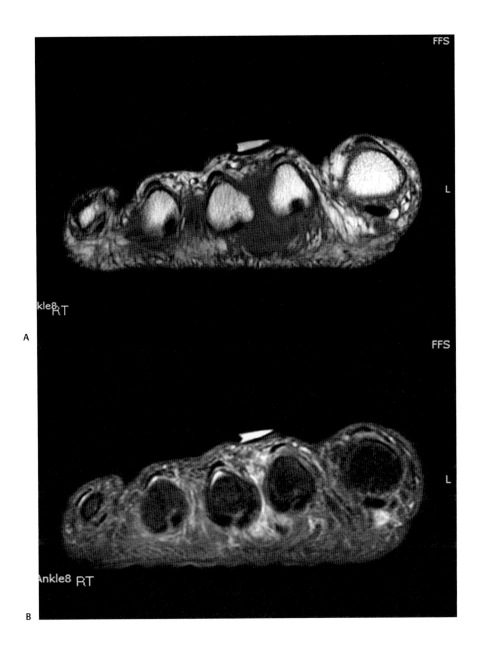

■ Clinical Presentation

A middle-aged female presents with swelling, fullness, and pain over the dorsal forefoot between the second and third metatarsal heads.

■ Imaging Findings

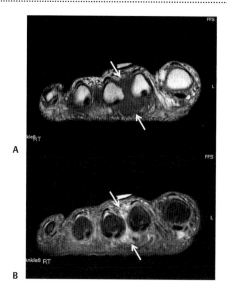

A

B

(A, B) Coronal fat-sensitive and fluid-sensitive MR images at the level of the metatarsal heads demonstrate a dumbbell-shaped hypointense T1, heterogeneous hyperintense T2 mixed solid and cystic mass between the second and third metatarsals (*arrows*). A dorsal soft tissue marker is in place at this site.

■ Differential Diagnosis

- ***Morton's neuroma:*** A nonneoplastic, perineural, fibrotic process centered around the plantar nerves of the forefoot between the metatarsal heads is consistent with this diagnosis. MRI reveals regional soft tissue fullness in these areas with heterogeneous hypointense T1 and hyperintense T2 signal.
- *Ganglion cyst:* A juxta-articular or juxtatendinous cystic focus of myxomatous/mucoid degeneration exhibiting relatively homogeneous hyperintense T2 and hypointense T1 signal.

■ Essential Facts

- Morton's neuroma represents a nonneoplastic, fibrous proliferative process centered around the plantar digital nerves of the forefoot.
- The typical patient is a middle-aged female with a history of poor-fitting shoes, typically high-heeled with a narrow toe box, resulting in entrapment of the plantar nerves between the metatarsal heads.
- Patients present with pain and numbness at the site of entrapment.
- Lesions typically exhibit low T1 and intermediate-high T2 signal intensity on MR imaging.
- Intermetatarsal bursal fluid distention of > 3 mm may be seen dorsal to these lesions.

■ Other Imaging Findings

- Ultrasound imaging may demonstrate a hypoechoic, interdigital mass possibly showing continuity with the plantar digital nerve.

✓ Pearls and ✗ Pitfalls

- ✓ Morton's neuromas most commonly occur in the second and third intermetatarsal spaces.
- ✗ Many patients with Morton's neuromas are asymptomatic.

Case 45

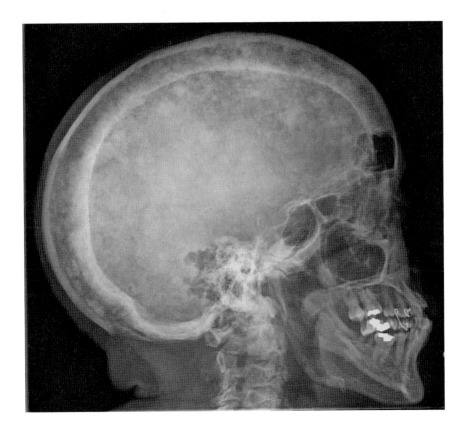

■ Clinical Presentation

A patient presents with elevation of serum alkaline phosphatase.

■ **Imaging Findings**

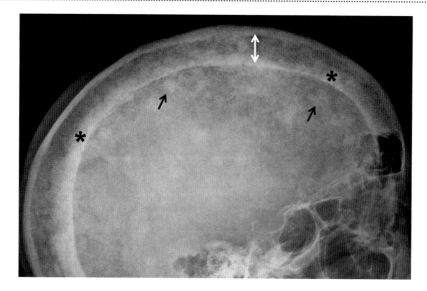

Lateral radiograph of the skull shows widening of the diploic space (*double white arrow*). There are several areas of focal rounded sclerosis (*black arrows*) resembling cotton wool. Marked thickening of the inner table of the skull (*asterisks*) is seen.

■ **Differential Diagnosis**

• ***Paget's disease:*** A mixed lytic and blastic benign bony disorder resulting in expansion of the diploic space of the skull with rounded sclerotic foci assuming a cotton wool appearance.
• *Metastasis:* Osteoblastic metastases may demonstrate a cotton wool appearance on skull radiographs. However, diffuse expansion of the diploic space is not a typical feature of this process.
• *Hyperostosis frontalis interna:* An entity typically seen in females which causes thickening of the inner table of the frontal bone.

■ **Essential Facts**

• Paget's disease of bone affects 3 to 4% of the population older than age 40 years.
• This disease predominantly involves the axial skeleton.
• Symptoms may include localized pain, tenderness, increased bone size, kyphosis of the spine, and decreased range of motion.
• Serum alkaline phosphatase is elevated secondary to an increased rate of bone formation.
• Urine hydroxyproline levels may be elevated.
• Paget's disease is composed of three phases which include the lytic, mixed, and blastic phases.
• The early or lytic phase of Paget's disease is characterized by osteolysis on radiographs.
• The vast majority of cases demonstrate mixed sclerotic/ lytic osseous changes resulting in characteristic radiographic findings of trabecular coarsening and cortical thickening.

• The blastic phase of this disease is responsible for the cotton wool appearance seen in the skull.
• Bone enlargement is particularly common in the blastic phase of Paget's disease.
• Disproportionate thickening of the inner table of the skull results in the "tam o'shanter" skull.

■ **Other Imaging Findings**

• Three-phase nuclear medicine bone scan demonstrates increased radiotracer uptake in all three stages of Paget's disease.
• MRI of Paget's disease demonstrates retention of the fat marrow signal intensity within the long bones, helping to distinguish this entity from a more aggressive malignant process.

✓ **Pearls and** ✗ **Pitfalls**

✓ Paget's disease is extremely rare in the ribs.
✓ Appendicular skeletal involvement is frequently unilateral.
✗ Nuclear medicine bone scan may underestimate the extent of Paget's disease.

Case 46

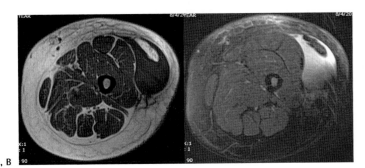

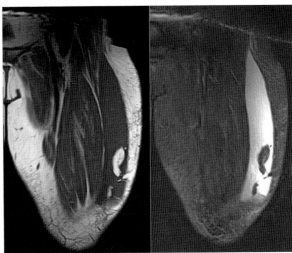

A, B

C, D

■ Clinical Presentation

A patient with a history of a motor vehicle accident 6 months prior presents with fullness over the lateral thigh.

■ **Imaging Findings**

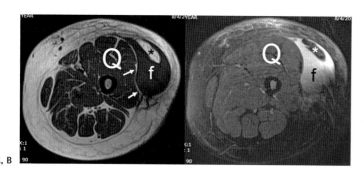

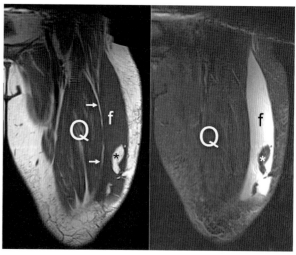

A, B   C, D

(A, B) Axial and **(C, D)** coronal fat-sensitive and fluid-sensitive MR images of the left thigh reveal a well-circumscribed subcutaneous low T1 and high T2 signal fluid collection (*f*). This collection is superficial to the lateral quadriceps muscles (*Q*), containing a lobule of internal fat signal (*asterisk*). A thin fat plane (*arrows*) lies at the interface of this lesion and the musculature.

■ **Differential Diagnosis**

- **Morel–Lavallée lesion (MLL):** A posttraumatic process resulting in a circumscribed, fluid signal intensity mass positioned between the muscle fascia and subcutaneous fat containing fat signal intensity lobules.
- *Myxoid neoplasm:* A simple or complex appearing mass with MR characteristics of complex fluid signal intensity with or without circumscribed borders exhibiting a complex internal enhancement pattern is consistent with this diagnosis.

■ **Essential Facts**

- MLL represents a posttraumatic internal degloving injury related to dehiscence of the muscle fascia from the subcutaneous fat secondary to a deceleration injury.
- The typical patient presentation is within weeks of the initial traumatic episode. Occasionally, patients present several months to years following the initial injury.
- This lesion is commonly associated with pelvic trauma and fractures.
- A potential space occurs along the plane of dehiscence accumulating fluid composed of serosanguineous fluid, blood products, necrotic fat, and/or lymphatic debris.
- MRI is the ideal imaging modality to characterize this lesion with the fluid collection demonstrating signal characteristics corresponding to blood products, serous fluid with or without sediment layers, and fat signal intensity lobules.
- Treatment may require percutaneous drainage with instillation of sclerosing agents to prevent recurrence.

■ **Other Imaging Findings**

- Ultrasound imaging may show hyperechoic nodules of internal fat surrounded by a hypoechoic or anechoic fluid collection.
- CT imaging may show fluid–fluid levels related to sediment with possible fat density lobules.

✓ **Pearls and ✗ Pitfalls**

✓ The most common location for this lesion is adjacent to the greater trochanter.
✓ A surrounding low-signal fibrous pseudocapsule is typically seen on MRI.
✗ Depending on the location, bursitis may have a similar appearance to MLL, complicating the diagnosis.

Case 47

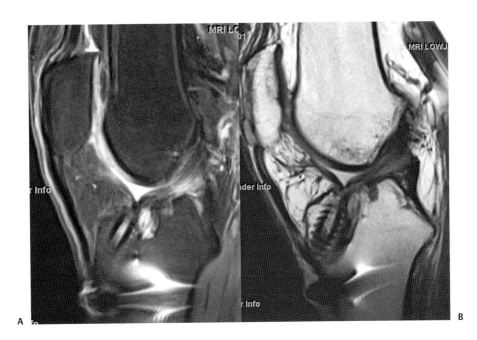

A   B

■ Clinical Presentation

A patient who is status post-anterior cruciate ligament (ACL) reconstruction presents with limited extension on physical exam.

■ **Imaging Findings**

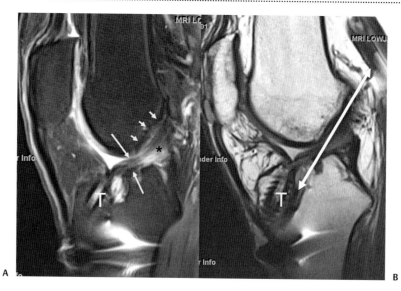

(A) Sagittal fluid-sensitive and **(B)** proton density MR imaging of the knee demonstrates an anterior cruciate ligament (ACL) graft in place. The tibial tunnel (*T*) is positioned anterior to the roof of the intercondylar notch (*small arrows*) as illustrated by the *double-headed arrow*. Abnormal signal intensity with posterior bowing (*asterisk*) are seen about the ACL graft mid-fibers. The distal ACL graft (*long arrows*) is incarcerated between the anterior margin of the intercondylar notch and the proximal tibia.

■ **Differential Diagnosis**

• *Anterior cruciate ligament graft impingement:* Anterior positioning of the tibial tunnel relative to the roof of the intercondylar notch resulting in posterior bowing of the ACL graft which contains intrasubstance MR signal increase are features of this diagnosis.

■ **Essential Facts**

• Positioning of the tibial tunnel during ACL reconstruction is crucial in preventing impingement of the graft against the roof of the intercondylar notch upon knee extension.
• ACL graft impingement, also referred to as roof impingement, occurs with anterior positioning of the tibial tunnel relative to the roof of the intercondylar notch.
• Patients may present with limited range of motion upon extension with pain.
• The roof of the intercondylar notch, also referred to as Blumensaat's line, may be extrapolated distally on lateral knee radiographs or sagittal MR images to verify tunnel positioning.
• The entire tibial osseous tunnel should be posterior and parallel to this line for optimal graft functioning.
• MR imaging may show posterior bowing of the ACL graft with anterior tunnel positioning.
• These patients are at risk for ACL graft degeneration and eventual ACL graft rupture.
• Treatment with notchplasty may increase ACL graft clearance for proper graft functioning.

■ **Other Imaging Findings**

• Full extension lateral knee radiographs will demonstrate anterior positioning of the tibial tunnel.

✓ **Pearls and ✗ Pitfalls**

✓ Abnormal MR signal intensity involving the anterior two thirds of the graft is typical for this form of impingement.
✗ Slight flexion of the knee during MR evaluation of the ACL graft may fail to adequately display tibial tunnel positioning.

Case 48

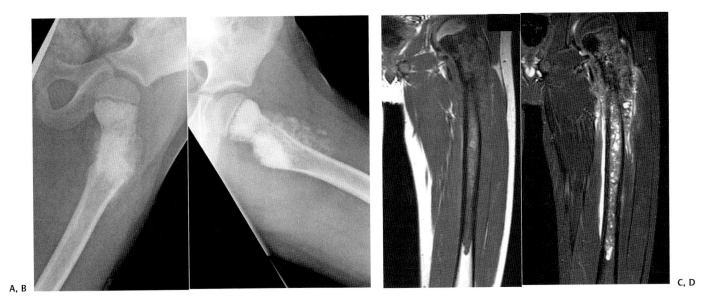

A, B

C, D

■ Clinical Presentation

A pediatric patient presents with localized left hip and thigh pain of several months' duration.

■ Imaging Findings

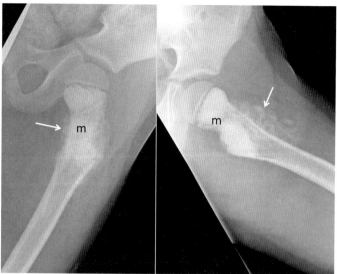
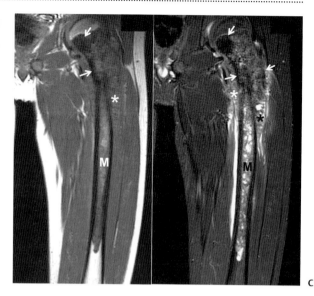

A, B

C, D

(A, B) Radiographs of the left hip demonstrate a proximal femoral metaphyseal medullary based osteoblastic mass (*m*) with soft tissue osteoid matrix (*arrows*). **(C, D)** Coronal fat-sensitive and fluid-sensitive MR imaging shows an intramedullary mass (*M*) involving the femoral metaphysis with extension into the diaphysis demonstrating low T1 and high T2 signal. A soft tissue component (*asterisk*) is evident. Regions of blastic intramedullary bone formation (*arrows*) are seen.

■ Differential Diagnosis

- **Conventional osteosarcoma:** A primary malignant bone-forming lesion of the adolescent skeleton presenting in the femoral diametaphysis as an osteoblastic medullary-based mass with a soft tissue lesion.
- *Chronic osteomyelitis:* Cortical thickening, chronic appearing periosteal bone formation with a superimposed central lucent nidus or sinus track demonstrating hyperintense T2 signal on MR imaging are representative of this infectious process.

■ Essential Facts

- Conventional osteosarcoma is a primary malignant bone-forming tumor characterized by the production of osteoid or immature bone by malignant cells.
- This malignancy represents the most common primary bone tumor of adolescents and young adults, with a peak incidence between 13 and 16 years of age.
- Patients may present with pain and swelling.
- Although numerous variants of osteosarcoma exist, intramedullary conventional osteosarcoma represents 90% of all cases.
- Radiographs typically demonstrate an aggressive-appearing lesion with a broad zone of transition, cortical interruption, periosteal reaction with a Codman triangle, and osteoid matrix.
- The osteoid matrix may be detectable on radiographs and/or CT.

- MRI is ideal for assessing bony and soft tissue involvement with radionuclide bone scanning utilized for identifying metastasis.
- Treatment includes chemotherapy and surgery, with an increased serum lactate dehydrogenase (LDH) associated with poorer outcomes.

■ Other Imaging Findings

- Pulmonary metastasis from osteosarcoma may manifest as a spontaneous pneumothorax.

✓ Pearls and ✗ Pitfalls

- ✓ The most common locations for osteosarcoma include the metaphyses of long bones, particularly the distal femur, proximal tibia, and proximal humerus.
- ✗ Radiographic diagnosis of lytic osteosarcomas may be challenging given decreased or absent osteoid mineralization.

Case 49

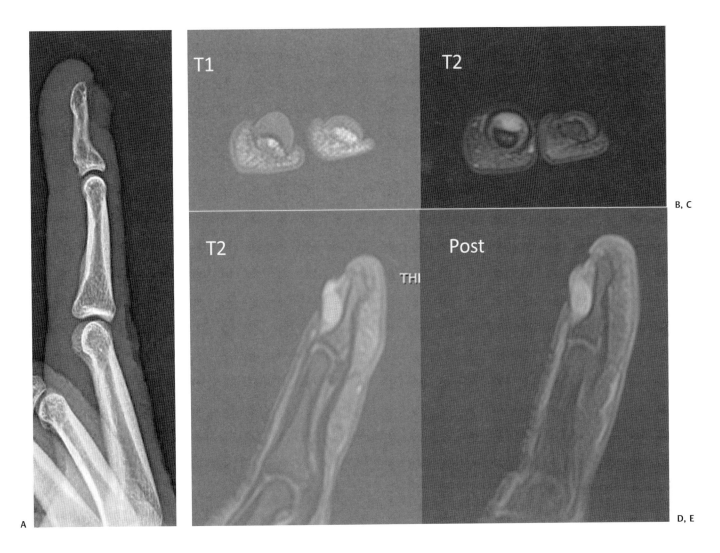

A

T1

T2

B, C

T2

THI

Post

D, E

■ **Clinical Presentation**

A 45-year-old female patient presents with several months' history of ring-finger pain.

■ Imaging Findings

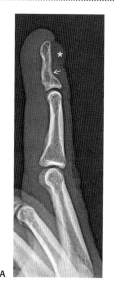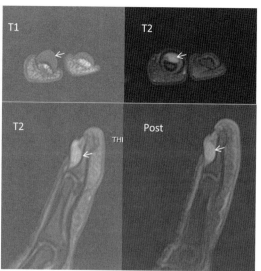

(A) Lateral radiograph of the ring finger demonstrates focal soft tissue fullness elevating the nail bed (*asterisk*). There is extrinsic cortical remodeling of the dorsal margin of the distal phalanx (*arrow*). **(B–E)** Axial fat-sensitive and fluid-sensitive MR images along with sagittal fluid-sensitive and post-gadolinium MR images demonstrate a circumscribed, ovoid hypointense T1, hyperintense T2 homogeneously enhancing lesion (*arrows*). This lesion abuts the distal phalanx dorsal cortex and is intimately associated with the nail bed.

■ Differential Diagnosis

- **Glomus tumor:** A painful soft tissue mass arising from the glomus cell typically seen in the nail bed.
- *Ganglion cyst:* A juxta-articular degenerative cyst typically associated with the distal interphalangeal joint of the finger.
- *Epidermoid inclusion cyst:* A posttraumatic, painless intra-osseous lesion resulting from penetrating trauma frequently seen in the distal phalanges.

■ Essential Facts

- A glomus tumor represents a neoplasm of the glomus cell.
- The glomus cell regulates blood flow between arterioles and venules containing a rich nerve supply. The glomus cell also provides a role in thermoregulation.
- These features of the glomus cell are responsible for the typical patient presentation of focal fingertip pain, tenderness, and sensitivity to cold.
- This lesion is more commonly seen in females within the 3rd to 4th decades of life.
- Symptoms may be present for several months or even years.
- The chronicity of these lesions is responsible for the radiographic findings of chronic extrinsic cortical remodeling and cystic change within the distal phalanges.

- Typical MRI features are a hypointense T1, hyperintense T2 soft tissue mass demonstrating avid enhancement.
- Glomus tumor is typically a solitary lesion, although multifocal lesions have been reported.
- Complete surgical excision is curative.

■ Other Imaging Findings

- Ultrasound imaging may show a solid hypoechoic mass deep to the nail bed with increased color Doppler flow.

✓ Pearls and ✗ Pitfalls

✓ The hypervascular nature of this lesion manifests with avid homogeneous post-gadolinium enhancement on MRI and increased color Doppler flow on ultrasound imaging.

✗ Glomus tumors > 1.5 cm tend to appear more heterogeneous on fluid-sensitive MR imaging and may demonstrate non-uniform enhancement, complicating the diagnosis.

✗ Lesions < 2 to 3 mm may be difficult to detect on MR imaging.

Case 50

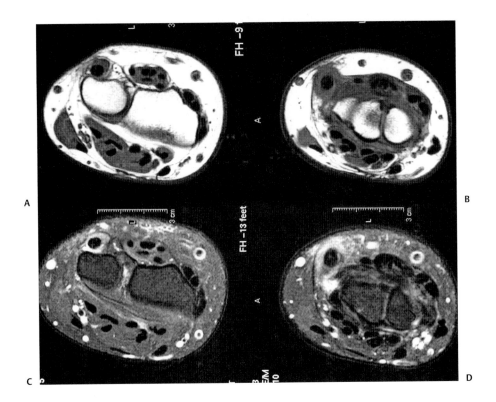

■ Clinical Presentation

A young adult patient presents with ulnar-sided wrist pain.

■ Imaging Findings

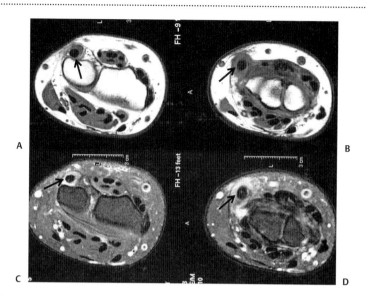

(A–D) Axial fat-sensitive and fluid-sensitive MR images through the wrist reveal fluid and synovial thickening surrounding a thickened extensor carpi ulnaris tendon (*arrows*). Minimal interstitial signal increase is seen within the enlarged tendon on the fluid-sensitive sequences.

■ Differential Diagnosis

- ***Extensor carpi ulnaris tenosynovitis/tendinopathy:***
  MR imaging demonstrating focal extensor carpi ulnaris (ECU) tendon enlargement with intratendinous signal increase with surrounding fluid and synovial thickening are features consistent with this diagnosis.
- *de Quervain's tenosynovitis:* Focal enlargement of the first extensor compartment tendons with surrounding soft tissue inflammatory changes including tenosynovitis are consistent with this diagnosis.

■ Essential Facts

- The ECU tendon occupies the sixth extensor compartment.
- Patients with ECU tendinopathy and tenosynovitis typically present with ulnar-sided wrist pain.
- Tendinopathy and tenosynovitis of this compartment is the second most common site of tendon disease in the wrist of athletes and results from repetitive microtrauma and/or overuse.
- Early changes of rheumatoid arthritis may manifest as ECU tendinopathy and tenosynovitis.
- Typical MRI findings of ECU tendinopathy include tendon thickening with increased signal on both T1- and T2-weighted images. Surrounding hyperintense T2 fluid signal within the tendon sheath is consistent with tenosynovitis.
- Traumatic injuries to the ECU tendon may lead to dislocation of the tendon from the ulnar styloid groove.

■ Other Imaging Findings

- Ultrasound imaging will display enlargement of the tendon with internal hypoechoic changes corresponding to interstitial tearing. Surrounding sonolucent or hypoechoic fluid represents tenosynovitis.

✓ Pearls and ✗ Pitfalls

- ✓ Long-standing ECU tenosynovitis/tendinopathy may exhibit focal periosteal reaction and remodeling of the ulnar styloid on radiographs.
- ✗ The ECU may normally display mild dorsal displacement from the ulnar groove upon wrist supination and extension or mild volar displacement with pronation and wrist flexion.

Case 51

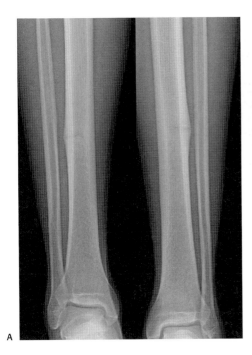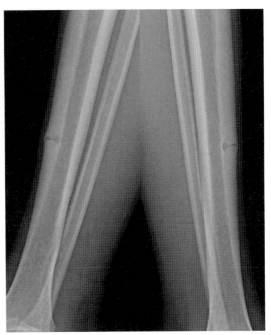

A

B

■ Clinical Presentation

A young adult runner presents with chronic bilateral leg pain.

■ Imaging Findings

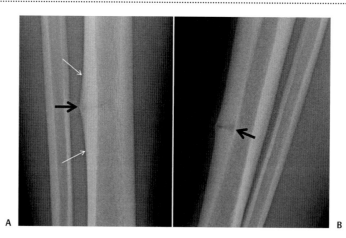

(A, B) Radiographs of the left and right tibia and fibula demonstrate transversely oriented lucencies (*black arrows*) extending through the anterior and lateral tibial cortices superimposed upon fusiform cortical thickening (*white arrows*).

■ Differential Diagnosis

- ***Tibial stress fractures:*** Bilateral mid-diaphyseal transversely oriented tibial cortical lucencies bordered by chronic cortical periosteal remodeling secondary to repetitive stresses applied to the healthy skeleton represent this diagnosis.

■ Essential Facts

- Stress fractures occur when normal bone is subjected to repetitive supraphysiologic stress.
- Osteoclastic resorption exceeds the rate of osteoblastic bone repair.
- This diagnosis should be considered in patients presenting with pain after a change in activity, especially if the activity is strenuous and the pain is in the lower extremities.
- Sequential radiographs demonstrate a spectrum of changes to include periosteal reaction, cortical hypertrophy, and/or a fracture lucency.
- Although transversely oriented tibial stress fractures are most common, longitudinally oriented cortical stress fractures may also occur.
- MRI is the modality of choice for detecting early tibial stress fractures, and correlates best with the severity of tibial stress injuries.

■ Other Imaging Findings

- Radionuclide bone scanning reveals isotope uptake in the area of stress injury and bony remodeling.

✓ Pearls and ✗ Pitfalls

- ✓ The medial cortical margin of the mid-diaphysis of the tibia is the favored site for stress injuries in the human skeleton.
- ✗ Radiographs are suboptimal for the early diagnosis of stress injuries.
- ✗ Symptoms from tibial stress injuries may be discordant with findings on radionuclide bone scan.

Case 52

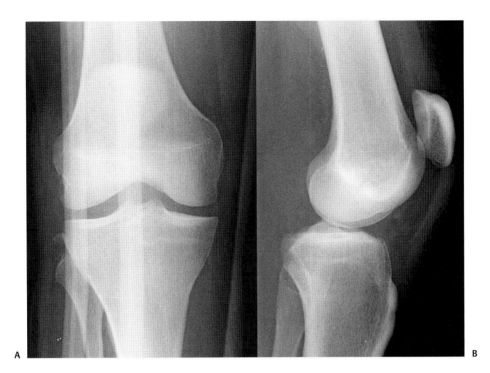

A   B

■ Clinical Presentation

A patient presents with trauma to the knee following a motor vehicle collision.

■ Further Work-up

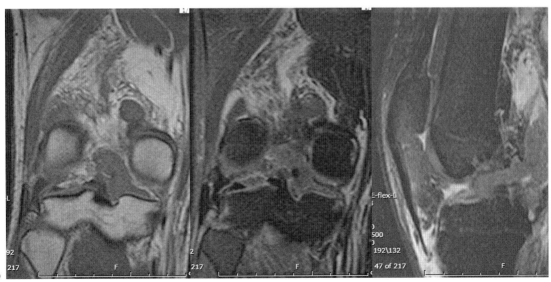

C, D   E

■ **Imaging Findings**

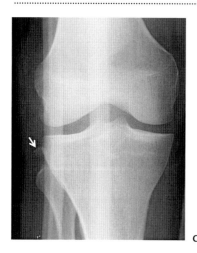
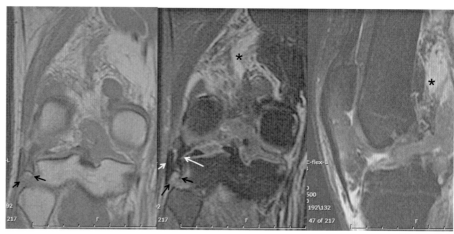

C   D, E

(A) Frontal radiograph of the knee demonstrates a horizontally oriented bony fragment (*white arrow*) positioned proximal to the fibular head. **(B–E)** Coronal fat-sensitive and fluid-sensitive MR images of the knee demonstrate an avulsion fracture fragment (*black arrows*) harvested from the fibular head attached to the biceps femoris tendon (*short white arrow*) and fibular collateral ligament (*long white arrow*). There is disruption of the cruciate ligaments demonstrated on sagittal fluid-sensitive MR images. Fluid and edema are seen along the posterior joint capsule (*asterisk*).

■ **Differential Diagnosis**

- *Arcuate sign:* A traumatic bony avulsion from the proximal fibula represented by a horizontally oriented fracture fragment associated with disruption of the biceps femoris tendon and fibular collateral ligament. This injury is associated with arcuate complex and cruciate ligament injuries.
- *Segond fracture:* A lateral tibial cortical capsular avulsion fracture with a high association with anterior cruciate ligament tears.

■ **Essential Facts**

- The arcuate sign derives its name from the horizontally oriented avulsion fracture fragment harvested from the fibular head at the site of the arcuate ligament complex.
- The arcuate ligament complex is comprised of the arcuate ligament, fibular collateral ligament, and popliteus muscle.
- Mechanism of injury involves a direct varus blow with the tibia in external rotation or a sudden hyperextension of the knee with the tibia internally rotated.
- Cruciate ligament tears from knee dislocation may coexist with this injury when severe.

■ **Other Imaging Findings**

- CT angiography may reveal popliteal vascular injury in the setting of knee dislocation.

✓ **Pearls and ✗ Pitfalls**

✓ MRI findings of fibular head contusion and severe popliteus muscle edema should raise suspicion for posterior lateral corner ligament injury.
✗ This bony avulsion may only be visualized on frontal knee radiographs.

Case 53

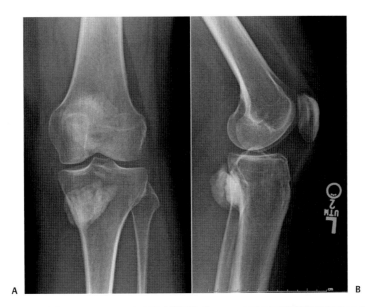

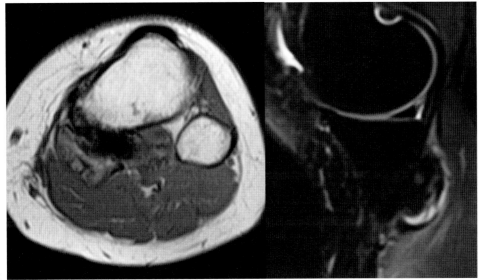

■ Clinical Presentation

A 30-year-old patient presents with chronic pain and fullness over the posterior knee.

■ Imaging Findings

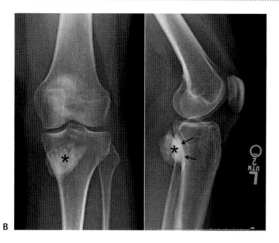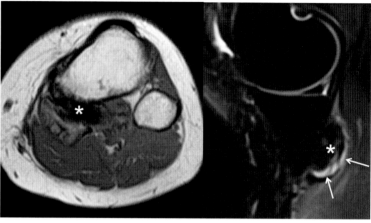

A, B   C, D

(A, B) Knee radiographs display a "mushroom-like" lobulated ossific mass (*asterisk*) arising from the posterior proximal tibial cortex with a broad-based stalk (*arrows*). **(C, D)** Axial fat-sensitive and sagittal fluid-sensitive MR images through this mass (*asterisk*) show persistent signal loss related to dense osteoid mineralization with no medullary extension of the lesion. A thin circumferential hyperintense T2 soft tissue mass (*arrows*) encircles the osteoid mass.

■ Differential Diagnosis

- ***Parosteal osteosarcoma:*** A surface variant of osteosarcoma represented by an osteoblastic cortical-based mass enclosed by a soft tissue mass characteristically seen in the 3rd through 4th decades of life.
- *Osteochondroma:* The most common benign bony lesion in an adult represented by a sessile or pedunculated osseous excrescence contiguous with the medullary canal containing a hyperintense T2 signal cartilaginous cap on MRI with or without chondroid calcifications.
- *Myositis ossificans:* A posttraumatic intramuscular mass demonstrating peripheral ossification with central soft tissue/fluid.

■ Essential Facts

- Parosteal osteosarcoma is the most common of the surface osteosarcomas.
- Peak incidence is in the 3rd and 4th decades with a female predominance.
- Patients may present with pain, swelling, and a palpable mass.
- This lesion involves the metaphysis of long tubular bones.
- This tumor is heavily mineralized and grows in an exophytic fashion from the outer layer of the cortex.

- A peripheral rim of immature bone formation manifests as a soft tissue mass.
- Radiographic findings include a rounded and/or lobulated ossific mass abutting the cortical surface of long bones.
- A radiolucent cleavage plane may be present between the cortex of the affected tubular bone and the lobulated osteoid component of the mass.
- MRI is ideal for assessing the peripheral soft tissue mass and any medullary bony extension.
- Low-grade lesions are usually treated with surgical resection requiring no neoadjuvant chemotherapy or radiation.

■ Other Imaging Findings

- Radionuclide bone scan will exhibit increased radiotracer uptake in the region of the ossified mass.

✓ Pearls and ✗ Pitfalls

✓ This lesion commonly affects the posterior aspect of the distal femoral metaphysis.

✗ Distinguishing parosteal osteosarcoma from other surface osteosarcoma variants may be difficult with radiographs alone.

Case 54

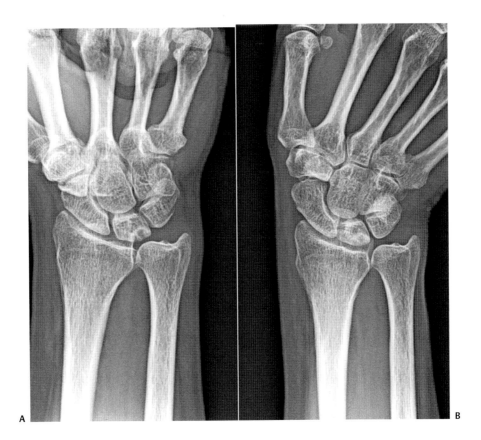

■ Clinical Presentation

A patient presents with chronic ulnar-sided wrist pain.

■ Imaging Findings

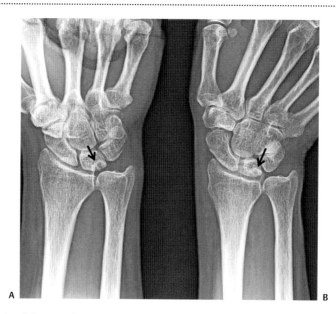

(A, B) Frontal and oblique radiographs of the wrist demonstrate ulnar plus variance. Mixed cystic and sclerotic changes lie within the proximal medial articular surface of the lunate (*arrows*).

■ Differential Diagnosis

- ***Ulnar impaction:*** A degenerative process associated with ulnar plus variance with adjacent proximal medial lunate cystic and sclerotic changes in a patient complaining of ulnar-sided wrist pain.
- *Kienböck's disease:* Osteonecrosis of the lunate demonstrating diffuse sclerosis on radiographs.

■ Essential Facts

- Ulnar impaction, also known as ulnar abutment, is a degenerative condition clinically manifested by ulnar-sided wrist pain.
- Premature bony contact/abutment occurs between the ulnar head and the lunate, typically seen with positive ulnar variance.
- Radiographic features include lunate and triquetral sclerosis and subcortical cyst formation.
- This condition may deteriorate to end-stage ulnar carpal osteoarthrosis.

■ Other Imaging Findings

- MRI demonstrates cartilage thinning at the ulnar lunate articulation with associated subcortical cyst formation and bone marrow edema.

✓ Pearls and ✗ Pitfalls

- ✓ Advanced changes of ulnar impaction may coexist with lunotriquetral ligament and triangular fibrocartilage tears.
- ✗ Ulnar impaction may be seen without anatomic variation in ulnar length.

Case 55

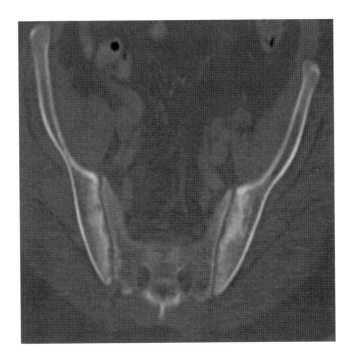

■ Clinical Presentation

A 42-year-old male patient presents with skin plaques and a history of low back pain.

■ **Imaging Findings**

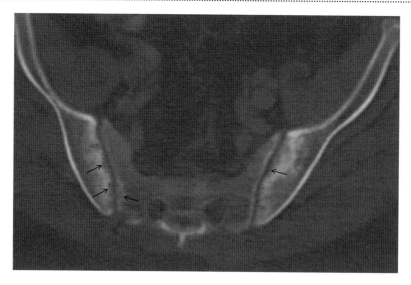

Axial CT image through the sacroiliac joints demonstrates asymmetric, periarticular sclerosis admixed with erosions (*arrows*), more notable along the iliac side of the articular margins.

■ **Differential Diagnosis**

- ***Psoriatic arthritis (PA):*** A seronegative spondyloarthropathy resulting in asymmetric erosive changes of the bilateral sacroiliac (SI) joints in conjunction with psoriatic skin plaques.
- *Ankylosing spondylitis:* A seronegative spondyloarthropathy causing symmetric SI joint erosions and eventual ankylosis without associated skin findings.
- *Septic arthritis:* A monoarticular infectious process which may be associated with periarticular fluid collections/abscess when involving the SI joint.

■ **Essential Facts**

- PA is a seronegative spondyloarthropathy that causes erosive and proliferative bony changes in the upper and lower extremities and axial skeleton.
- Sacroiliitis may represent the first osseous manifestation of the disease.
- PA sacroiliitis is usually bilateral and may be symmetric or asymmetric.
- Unlike ankylosing spondylitis, SI joint erosions are large.
- Spondylitis in PA is uncommon in the absence of sacroiliitis.
- CT findings of sacroiliitis are similar to findings on radiography and include erosions, sclerosis, and eventually ankylosis. CT is able to detect erosions along the subchondral bone plate at a much earlier stage of the disease in comparison to radiographs.

■ **Other Imaging Findings**

- Radionuclide bone scan exhibits increased uptake at the level of the SI joints related to the bony reparative process.
- MRI demonstrates bone marrow edema changes manifested by decreased T1 and increased T2 signal within the periarticular bone marrow of the SI joints.

✓ **Pearls and ✗ Pitfalls**

- ✓ The asymmetric SI joint features of PA allow distinction from ankylosing spondylitis and enteropathic spondyloarthropathies.
- ✗ CT evaluation of the SI joints does not allow assessment of subchondral or periarticular bone marrow edema.

Case 56

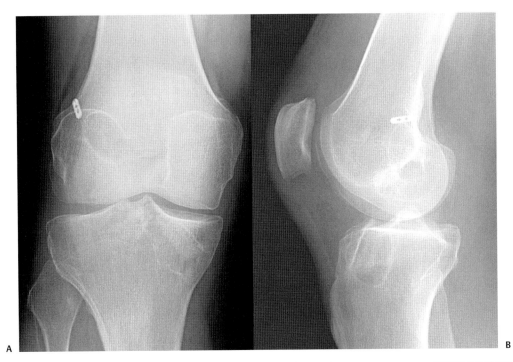

A

B

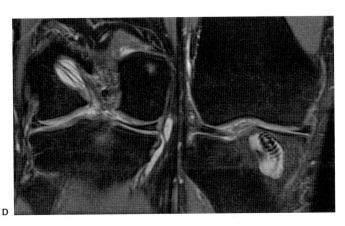

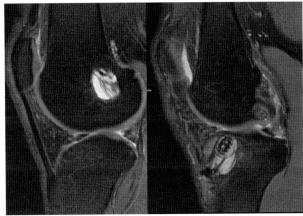

C, D

E, F

▪ Clinical Presentation

A patient presents with a remote history of anterior cruciate ligament (ACL) reconstruction with abnormality seen on radiographs.

■ Imaging Findings

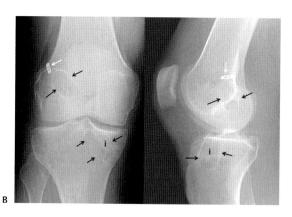

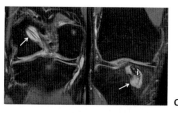

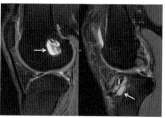

A, B

C, D

E, F

(A, B) Frontal and lateral radiographs of the knee demonstrate changes of ACL repair with a fixation button (*white arrow*) along the lateral femoral epicondyle. Cystic expansion of osseous tunnels (*black arrows*) is seen. A faintly opaque threaded interference screw (*i*) within the proximal tibia is present. **(C, D)** Coronal and **(E, F)** sagittal fluid-sensitive MR images demonstrate hyperintense T2 cystic expansion of the femoral and tibial tunnels (*white arrows*). The tibial interference screw (*i*) is surrounded by these cystic changes.

■ Differential Diagnosis

- ***Anterior cruciate ligament graft osseous tunnel cysts:*** Radiographic findings of prominent femoral and tibial tunnel expansile lucencies with corresponding MRI T2 cystic changes are compatible with this diagnosis.

■ Essential Facts

- ACL tunnel cyst formation is a complication of ACL reconstruction.
- Proposed etiologies for these cystic changes include necrosis, foreign body reaction, incomplete graft osseous integration, and extravasation of synovial fluid.
- MR and radiographic imaging characteristics include cystic widening of the osseous tunnels.
- Continued cystic fluid formation may result in eventual dissection into the ACL graft, causing splaying of the graft fibers.
- Eventual fluid extension may occur through the distal tibial osseous tunnel into the pretibial soft tissues with patients presenting with a pretibial soft tissue mass.

✓ Pearls and ✗ Pitfalls

- ✓ Femoral tunnel cysts are less common than tibial tunnel cysts.
- ✗ ACL graft tunnel cystic changes may normally be seen during the first year following ACL reconstruction with eventual resorption.

Case 57

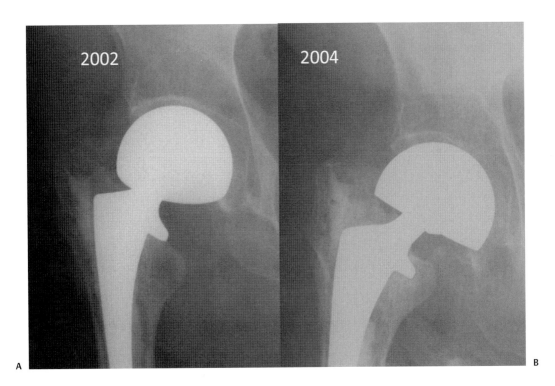

A

B

■ Clinical Presentation

A patient with a remote history of hip arthroplasty presents with chronic hip pain.

■ Imaging Findings

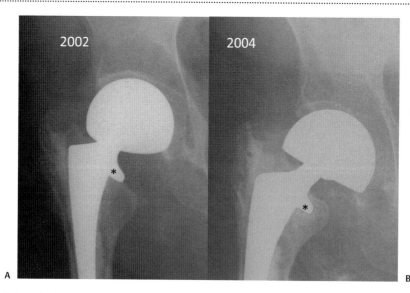

(A, B) Serial radiographs of the right hip demonstrate hemiarthroplasty changes with a cemented femoral prosthesis. The most recent radiograph (B) demonstrates sliding of the cemented femoral prosthesis (*asterisk*) into the medullary canal.

■ Differential Diagnosis

- **Hardware subsidence:** Progressive settling of the femoral component of hip arthroplasty by > 5 to 10 mm seen 1 to 2 years following the date of surgery is consistent with this diagnosis.

■ Essential Facts

- Hip and knee arthroplasty represent the most commonly performed joint arthroplasties in the human population.
- The femoral prosthesis may demonstrate normal vertical settling, or subsidence, into the femoral medullary canal of < 10 mm in the 1st year following hip arthroplasty.
- Subsidence occurring beyond this time interval is considered abnormal.
- Serial comparison radiographs must be utilized to detect significant changes of subsidence.
- Other associated radiographic findings include development of periprosthetic femoral lucency > 2 mm or a fracture through the cemented mantle of the femoral component.

■ Other Imaging Findings

- Radionuclide bone scan will show increased radiotracer uptake at the fracture sites.

✓ Pearls and ✗ Pitfalls

- ✓ Radiographic positioning of the medial femoral prosthetic collar relative to the adjacent lesser trochanter of the femur enables early detection of subsidence.
- ✗ Femoral prosthetic subsidence may be difficult to diagnose if the entire femoral prosthesis is not imaged and/or appropriate radiographic positioning of the hip arthroplasty components is not achieved.

Case 58

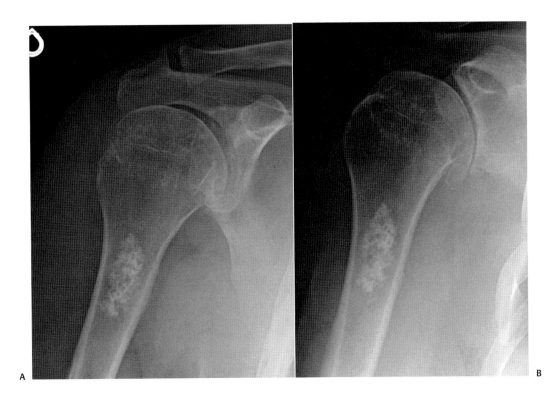

A

B

■ Clinical Presentation

A 65-year-old male patient presents with an incidental right shoulder lesion seen on preoperative chest X-ray.

■ Imaging Findings

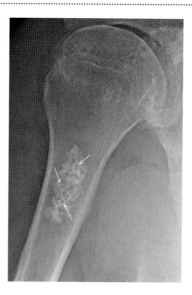

Frontal radiograph of the right shoulder demonstrates a lobulated cluster of densely calcified matrix containing "rings and arcs" (*arrows*) within the proximal humerus. No aggressive bony changes are seen.

■ Differential Diagnosis

- ***Enchondroma:*** A common benign medullary-based chondroid lesion demonstrating calcifications with "rings and arcs" morphology.
- *Bone infarct:* Intramedullary osteonecrosis characterized radiographically by a longitudinally oriented, serpentine calcific rim. This rim separates the necrotic and viable bone with no internal mineralization.

■ Essential Facts

- Enchondroma represents a benign neoplasm within the intramedullary bone arising from cartilage rests derived from the growth plate.
- This tumor represents the second most common benign chondroid tumor in the adult human skeleton, second to osteochondroma.
- Most enchondromas are diagnosed incidentally in the 3rd or 4th decades.
- These tumors are most commonly seen in the small bones of the hand.
- Classic radiographic findings include circumscribed lucent changes within the medullary canal of a long bone with mild endosteal scalloping.
- Chondroid calcifications appear as stippled or round/semicircular "ring and arc" calcifications.
- Proximal humeral enchondromas are typically discovered incidentally on shoulder MRI or chest X-ray.
- Transformation of a solitary enchondroma to chondrosarcoma is rare.

■ Other Imaging Findings

- CT imaging demonstrates replacement of the normal appendicular fatty marrow and trabeculae with a circumscribed lobulated soft tissue density. CT allows early detection of endosteal thinning and provides optimal characterization of the stippled or "ring and arc" calcifications.

✓ Pearls and ✗ Pitfalls

✓ Enchondroma is rare in the distal phalanges and carpal bones.

✗ Bone infarcts smaller than 1.5–2.0 cm may be indistinguishable from enchondroma on radiography.

Case 59

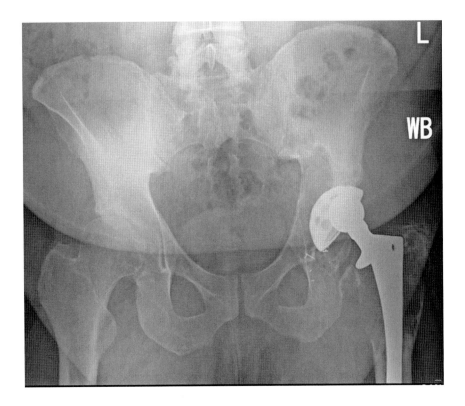

■ Clinical Presentation

A patient with a hip arthroplasty presents with worsening chronic hip pain and discomfort.

■ **Imaging Findings**

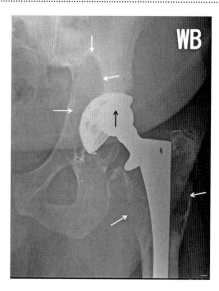

Single frontal radiograph of the pelvis demonstrates left hip noncemented total arthroplasty change. Extensive scalloped lucencies (*white arrows*) abut the acetabular and femoral components. The femoral head prosthesis shows superior migration (*black arrow*) within the acetabular cup.

■ **Differential Diagnosis**

• *Particle disease:* A noninfectious, inflammatory process seen with joint arthroplasties. Radiographs demonstrate aggressive, scalloped periprosthetic osteolysis with or without an eccentrically positioned femoral head component.
• *Hardware infection:* Osteomyelitis at the implant site of hardware demonstrated radiographically by ill-defined, shaggy perihardware lucencies.

■ **Essential Facts**

• Particle disease, also known as *aggressive granulomatosis*, is a histiocytic response within the bone driven by small polyethylene particles shed from the articular lining of orthopaedic hardware.
• Radiographs reveal localized, aggressive-appearing, scalloped regions of osteolysis along the bone hardware interface.
• Patients may be asymptomatic until the bony changes are extensive enough to cause mechanical loosening of the hardware.
• Abnormal polyethylene liner wear may be present and is demonstrated on radiographs by a superiorly malpositioned femoral head component.

■ **Other Imaging Findings**

• Lytic bony changes on MR imaging consist of intermediate signal intensity similar to, or slightly brighter than, skeletal muscle on both T1- and T2-weighted images.

✓ **Pearls and ✗ Pitfalls**

✓ Scalloped periprosthetic lucencies associated with particle disease seldom contain sclerotic margins.
✗ Residual degenerative subcortical cystic changes in the surrounding periprosthetic bone stock may mimic particle disease, emphasizing the use of comparison films.

Case 60

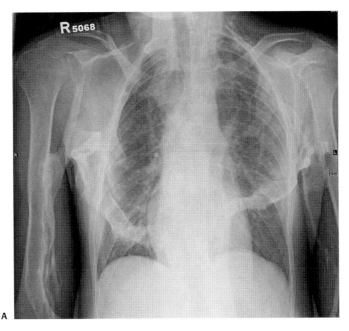

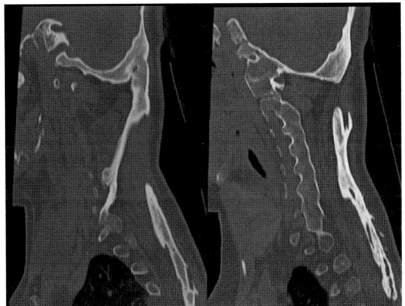

■ Clinical Presentation

A 25-year-old patient status post fall from a skateboard presents for trauma evaluation.

■ Imaging Findings

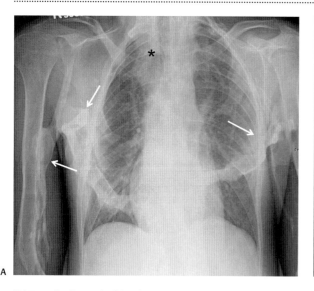

A

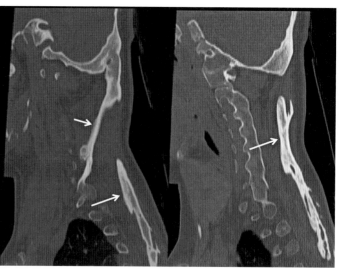

B, C

(A) Frontal radiograph of the chest shows extensive linear bone formation overlying the right humerus and bilateral hemithoraces (*arrows*). Dense opacification overlies the right paratracheal region (*asterisk*). **(B, C)** Sagittal reconstructed CT scans through the cervical spine demonstrate bulky linear ossification extending from the skull base to the posterior cervical spine (*short arrow*). A separate longitudinally oriented ossified mass is seen within the posterior cervical spine musculature (*long arrows*).

■ Differential Diagnosis

- **Fibrodysplasia ossificans progressiva (FOP):** A genetic condition associated with progressive and extensive deposits of heterotopic ossification accumulating around multiple joints.
- *Tumoral calcinosis:* A familial condition characterized by lobulated cloudlike calcific soft tissue deposits adjacent to the bursae of multiple joints.
- *Myositis ossificans:* Focal posttraumatic/reactive intramuscular bone formation most commonly seen adjacent to the humerus and femur.

■ Essential Facts

- FOP, previously known as *myositis ossificans progressiva*, represents a rare familial disorder characterized by progressive heterotopic ossification beginning in childhood.
- Ossification progresses in a cranial to caudal fashion in a periarticular distribution, eventually causing immobilization.
- Initial lesions usually occur in the back adjacent to the upper spine and shoulder girdle.
- Patients rarely survive beyond middle adulthood, with most dying in the 3rd or 4th decade secondary to pneumonia.
- Radiographs and CT reveal elongated and thickened regions of bridging ossification along the appendicular and axial skeleton.

■ Other Imaging Findings

- Radionuclide bone scan will show increased radiotracer uptake at the fracture sites.

✓ Pearls and ✗ Pitfalls

- ✓ Foot and hand radiographs may reveal short great toes and thumbs.
- ✗ Paralyzed patients may exhibit extensive periarticular heterotopic ossification resembling this disorder.

Case 61

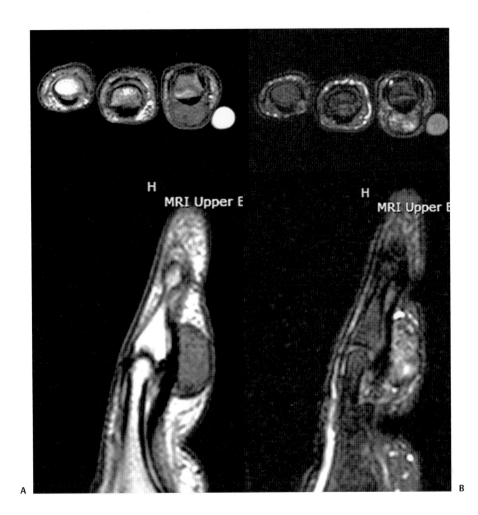

▪ Clinical Presentation

A 40-year-old female patient presents with a long-standing painless mass in her index finger.

■ **Imaging Findings**

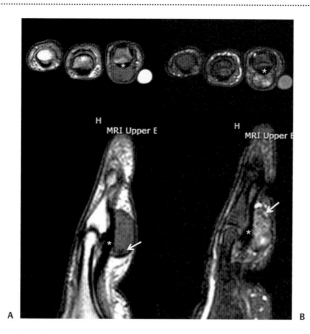

(A, B) Axial and sagittal fat- and fluid-sensitive MR imaging through the index finger displays a low-signal lobulated mass intimately associated with the flexor tendon (*asterisk*) with scattered internal regions of diminished T1/T2 signal (*arrows*).

■ **Differential Diagnosis**

- **Giant cell tumor (GCT) of the tendon sheath:** A synovial-based, benign, lobulated mass containing low T1/T2 MRI signal with a high affinity for the flexor tendons of the hand is characteristic of this lesion.
- *Fibroma of the tendon sheath:* A benign, solid fibrous lesion of the hand and foot which demonstrates intermediate to increased T2 and decreased T1 signal intensity on MRI.
- *Tophaceous gout:* A crystalline soft tissue mass associated with gout which demonstrates heterogeneous T1/T2 signal increase on MRI.

■ **Essential Facts**

- GCT of the tendon sheath is a nonmalignant proliferative disorder of the synovium characterized by cellular hemosiderin deposition causing low signal on MRI.
- This lesion is seen in the 3rd to 5th decades, with a slight female predominance.
- These masses arise from tendons, ligaments, or joint capsules of the hands and feet.

- GCT of the tendon sheath typically lies along the volar margin of the first three digits of the hand, most commonly the index and long fingers.
- These lesions are uncommon in the wrist.
- Some authorities classify fibromas and GCT tendon sheath along a spectrum of the same pathology.

■ **Other Imaging Findings**

- Hand radiographs demonstrate a dense, lobulated soft tissue mass which may cause underlying bony extrinsic erosive and/or cystic changes from mass effect.

✓ **Pearls and ✗ Pitfalls**

✓ This lesion typically demonstrates blooming artifact on gradient echo MRI related to hemosiderin deposition.
✗ GCT of the tendon sheath and fibroma of the tendon sheath may be indistinguishable on MRI in the absence of GCT hemosiderin deposition.

Case 62

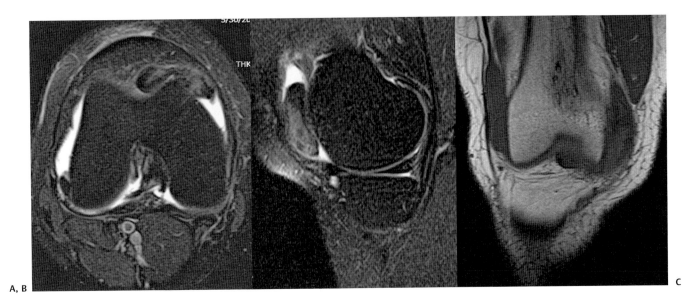

A, B

C

■ Clinical Presentation

A 45-year-old patient presents with knee pain.

■ Imaging Findings

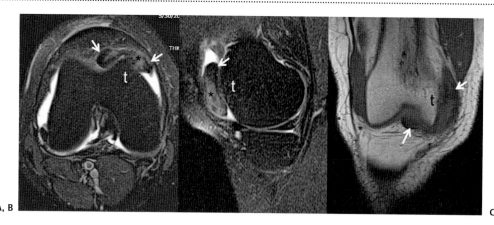

A, B   C

(A, B) Axial and sagittal fluid-sensitive and **(C)** coronal fat-sensitive MR images through the anterior knee joint show overall decreased signal intensity of an intra-articular soft tissue mass (*arrows*). This mass is draped over the medial trochlea (*t*) of the distal femur, with a surrounding small joint effusion.

■ Differential Diagnosis

- ***Focal pigmented villonodular synovitis (PVNS):*** A benign synovial-based, hemosiderin-rich mass lesion demonstrating low T1 and T2 signal intensity on MRI.
- *Loose osseous cartilaginous body (synovial osteochondromatosis):* A primary or degenerative joint-based osseous and/or chondral body exhibiting intermediate to increased T1 and T2 signal on MRI.
- *Synovial hemangioma:* A synovial-based vascular lesion associated with serpentine vascular channels and phleboliths, commonly seen in the knee, which may cause intra-articular hemorrhage with synovial hemosiderin deposition.

■ Essential Facts

- Focal PVNS is seen in young adults between the 3rd and 4th decades of life.
- The knee is the most frequently involved joint, particularly the infrapatellar fat.
- Focal PVNS is represented by focal benign proliferation of synovial tissue with intracellular deposition of hemosiderin accounting for the low T1/T2 MR signal characteristics.
- Hemosiderin deposition is accentuated with gradient echo MR imaging.
- This solitary lobulated intra-articular soft tissue mass reveals avid post-gadolinium enhancement on MRI.
- No malignant potential exists and treatment is local synovectomy.

■ Other Imaging Findings

- Three-phase nuclear medicine bone scan demonstrates increased uptake on the blood flow and blood pool phases.

✓ Pearls and ✗ Pitfalls

- ✓ Calcifications on radiography exclude this diagnosis.
- ✗ Localized intra-articular PVNS is usually not detectable on radiography.

Case 63

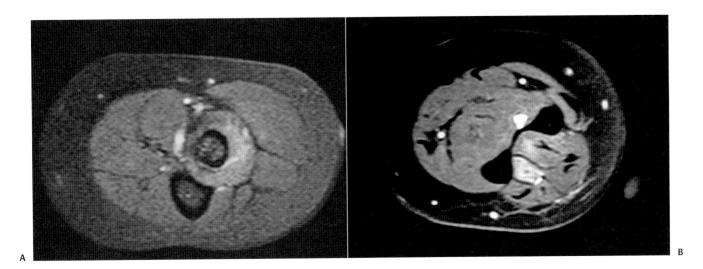

A   B

■ Clinical Presentation

A patient presents with forearm pain and weakness.

■ **Imaging Findings**

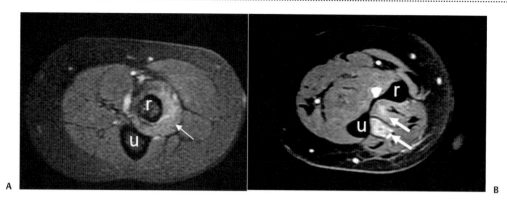

(A, B) Axial fluid-sensitive MR images through the elbow and proximal forearm, radius (*r*), and ulna (*u*) demonstrate geographic increased signal intensity within the supinator muscle (*thin arrow*) and within the proximal forearm extensor musculature (*thick arrows*).

■ **Differential Diagnosis**

- ***Posterior interosseous nerve syndrome:*** An entrapment neuropathy involving the posterior motor branch of the radial nerve resulting in geographic neurogenic muscle edema localized to the supinator and proximal forearm extensor musculature.
- *Muscle strain:* A traumatic muscle injury manifested on MRI as muscular edema with or without architectural muscle fiber disruption in a haphazard pattern. Surrounding soft tissue fluid signal intensity is typically present.

■ **Essential Facts**

- Posterior interosseous nerve syndrome represents an entrapment neuropathy involving the motor branch of the radial nerve, the posterior interosseous nerve, at the level of the supinator muscle.
- This entity is also referred to as *supinator syndrome* or *deep radial syndrome*.
- Compression of the nerve occurs most commonly along the tendinous proximal edge of the supinator muscle.
- This site of compression is typically in the region of the arcade of Frohse, a congenital fibrous adhesion between the brachialis and brachioradialis, present in ~30 to 50% of the population.

- Less common causes of extrinsic nerve compression result from radial head fractures, local tumors, ectatic blood vessels, or intracapsular elbow pathology.
- The typical presentation is forearm pain and weakness.
- Diagnosis is based on the muscle denervation pattern displayed on MRI with geographic muscle edema observed in the acute/subacute phase of denervation and muscle atrophy seen with chronic denervation.
- Muscle involvement includes the supinator and extensor musculature.

■ **Other Imaging Findings**

- Ultrasound imaging may reveal a hypoechoic and swollen posterior interosseous nerve.

✓ **Pearls and ✗ Pitfalls**

✓ This entrapment neuropathy spares the extensor carpi radialis muscle belly.
✗ Direct MRI visualization of structural compression on the posterior interosseous nerve is seldom possible.

Case 64

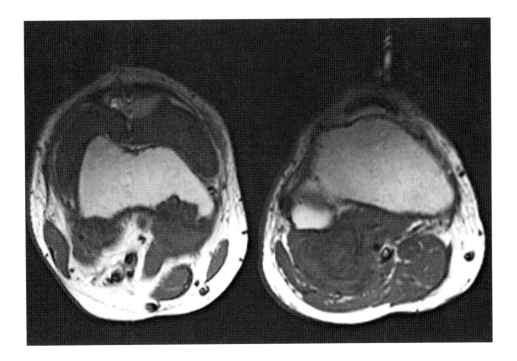

■ Clinical Presentation

MR evaluation of the knee with artifact.

■ **Imaging Findings**

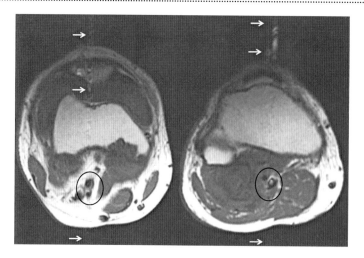

Axial fat-sensitive MR images through the knee joint demonstrate artifact (*arrows*) aligned along the Y-axis originating from the popliteal artery (*encircled*).

■ **Differential Diagnosis**

• ***Pulsation artifact:*** Artifactual signal created from the pulsation of vascular structures which occurs at regular intervals aligned along the Y-axis, or phasing encoding direction, as seen on this axial knee MRI.

■ **Essential Facts**

• Arterial vascular motion leads to reproduction of the moving vascular structure (ghosting artifact) in an abnormal but predictable position within the plane of imaging.
• Pulsation artifact is reproduced along the phase encoding direction.
• This pulsation artifact is reproduced at constant intervals.

✓ **Pearls and ✗ Pitfalls**

✓ Pulsation artifact may be resolved by utilizing electrocardiogram gating, saturation pulses, or gradient moment nulling.
✗ Inability to recognize this artifact may cause erroneous assignment of pathology to otherwise normal structures.

Case 65

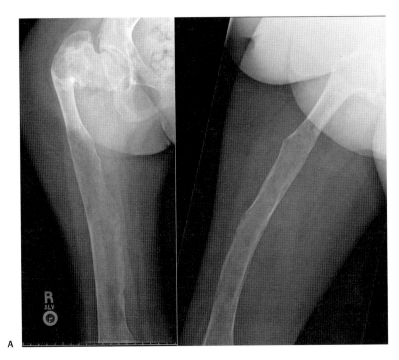 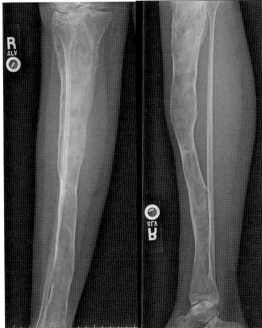

A   B

■ Clinical Presentation

A young adult patient presents with bony deformities.

■ **Imaging Findings**

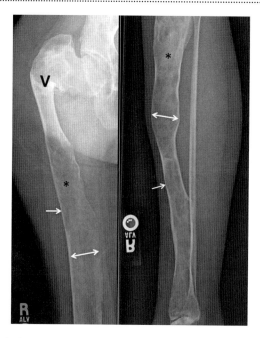

Radiographs of the right femur, tibia, and fibula demonstrate a varus deformity involving the proximal femur (*V*) representative of a shepherd's crook deformity. Anterior and lateral bowing of the tibial diaphysis is seen. Diffuse intramedullary "ground-glass" matrix (*asterisk*) is seen with overexpansion of the medullary canals (*double arrows*). Marked cortical endosteal thinning (*thin arrows*) is seen along the femoral and tibial diaphyses.

■ **Differential Diagnosis**

• ***Fibrous dysplasia (polyostotic):*** Multifocal fibrous marrow replacement centered in the diametaphyseal regions of the long bones causing medullary expansion with a hazy ground-glass appearance are characteristic of this process. Associated proximal femoral shepherd's crook deformity along with anterior bowing of the tibia further support this diagnosis.

■ **Essential Facts**

• Fibrous dysplasia represents a bone disorder characterized by overgrowth of marrow fibro-osseous tissue which accounts for the ground-glass or "smoky" appearance seen on radiographs.
• Patients present at approximately 8 years of age secondary to pain, limp, or pathologic fracture.
• Females are affected slightly more often than males.
• Lesions can occur in any bone but favor the femur and tibia.
• Proximal femoral varus deformity is known as shepherd's crook deformity related to abnormal remodeling from altered biomechanics across this region.
• Monostotic and polyostotic variants of this disease process are seen.
• Approximately 20 to 30% of cases are polyostotic.
• This disease typically becomes quiescent at puberty.

■ **Other Imaging Findings**

• MRI signal characteristics of fibrous dysplasia are variable and may exhibit decreased T1 and T2 signal representing fibrous tissue. Other MR signal changes may include hyperintense T2 cystic change or fluid–fluid levels.

✓ **Pearls and ✗ Pitfalls**

✓ Periosteal reaction should not be seen with fibrous dysplasia except in the presence of fracture or malignant degeneration.
✗ A separate and distinct lesion arising from the tibial cortex, osteofibrous dysplasia, may resemble fibrous dysplasia.

Case 66

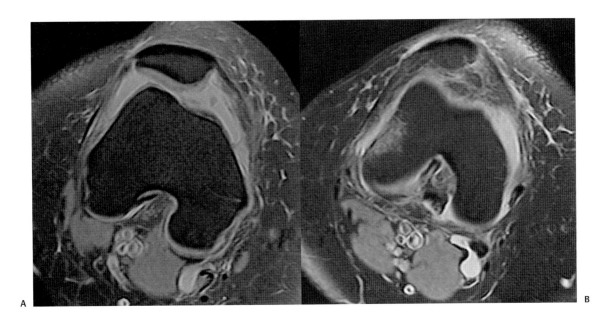

A   B

■ **Clinical Presentation**

A 25-year-old female patient presents with a twisting injury to the knee.

■ Imaging Findings

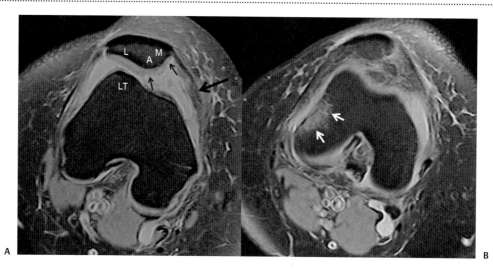

(A, B) Axial fluid-sensitive MR images through the patellofemoral compartment demonstrate a moderate-sized effusion. There is lateral subluxation of the patella with lateral overhanging of the lateral patellar facet (*L*) relative to the lateral trochlea (*LT*). Subcortical bone marrow edema is present along the periphery of the lateral femoral condyle (*short white arrows*). Cartilage irregularity (*short black arrows*) involves the patellar apex (*A*), and medial patellar facet (*M*). There is thickening with signal increase within the mid-fibers of the medial patellofemoral retinaculum (*long black arrow*).

■ Differential Diagnosis

• ***Patellofemoral dislocation (lateral):*** Bone bruising and/or fracture of the lateral femoral condyle and medial patella with residual lateral patellar translation and medial patellofemoral retinacular injury are diagnostic of this dislocation.

■ Essential Facts

• Lateral patellofemoral dislocation typically occurs from a flexed knee with internal rotation on a planted foot with a valgus component.
• The typical patient is a female in the second decade of life.
• MRI may be utilized to diagnose prior lateral patellofemoral dislocation.
• Typical findings on MRI include bone marrow edema/kissing contusions and/or fractures along the periphery of the lateral femoral condyle and the medial patellar facet.

• Additional findings may include adjacent curvilinear bony fragments, medial patellar facet/patellar apex chondral loss, medial patellofemoral retinacular disruption or sprain, lateral patellofemoral subluxation, and a joint effusion.
• Approximately 50% of patients who are managed conservatively following a first-time lateral patellofemoral dislocation will experience subsequent patellofemoral dislocations.

✓ Pearls and ✗ Pitfalls

✓ Axial radiographs of the patellofemoral joint may demonstrate curvilinear ossific debris adjacent to the lateral femoral condyle or patellar facets.
✗ A large joint effusion and/or hyperextension of the knee may cause nonpathologic, mild lateral patellar subluxation.

Case 67

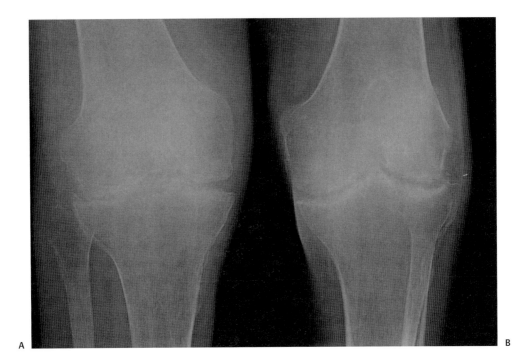

A   B

■ Clinical Presentation

A middle-aged female patient presents with polyarthralgias.

■ Imaging Findings

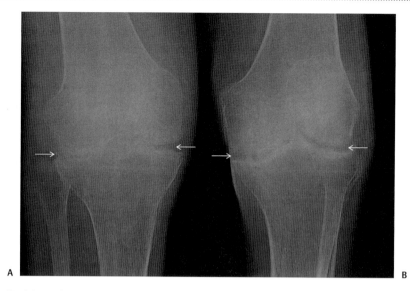

(A, B) Frontal radiograph of both knees demonstrates marked osteopenia. Symmetric narrowing of the medial and lateral compartments is seen with erosive changes involving the subchondral bone at the level of the tibial plateaus and femoral condyles (*arrows*). No significant osteophyte formation is present.

■ Differential Diagnosis

- **Rheumatoid arthritis (RA):** A symmetric and erosive inflammatory arthropathy resulting in narrowing of the bilateral knee joints with involvement of the medial and lateral femorotibial compartments in conjunction with osteopenia, subchondral erosions, and lack of osteophytes are characteristic of this diagnosis.
- *Osteoarthrosis:* A degenerative process characterized by medial femorotibial compartment joint space loss, subchondral sclerosis, and osteophytosis.
- *Septic arthritis:* Periarticular osteopenia, marginal erosions, and gradual joint space loss in a monoarticular distribution are consistent with this infectious arthropathy.

■ Essential Facts

- RA is a chronic, systemic polyarticular disease that predominantly involves synovial lined joints in a symmetric fashion.
- RA represents the most common inflammatory arthritis affecting the knee joints.
- Up to 13% of patients with RA present with the knee as the initial site of involvement.
- Inflammatory changes with synovial thickening and pannus formation are responsible for the radiographically detectable arthropathic changes.

- Symmetric knee involvement is common with radiographs demonstrating osteopenia and periarticular erosions which may progress to subarticular erosions.
- Equal loss of joint space along the medial and lateral femorotibial compartments is typical with overall paucity of osteophyte formation.
- Large subcortical periarticular cysts and erosive widening of the intercondylar notch may also be seen.

■ Other Imaging Findings

- Joint effusions and large Baker's cyst containing synovial thickening are characteristic findings seen on MR imaging.

✓ Pearls and ✗ Pitfalls

- ✓ Radiographic findings of bilateral and atraumatic knee joint effusions and periarticular osteopenia with diffuse and uniform femoral tibial joint space loss in a young adult female are highly suspicious for RA.
- ✗ Large isolated subcortical bony cysts from RA may mimic a lytic neoplasm.

Case 68

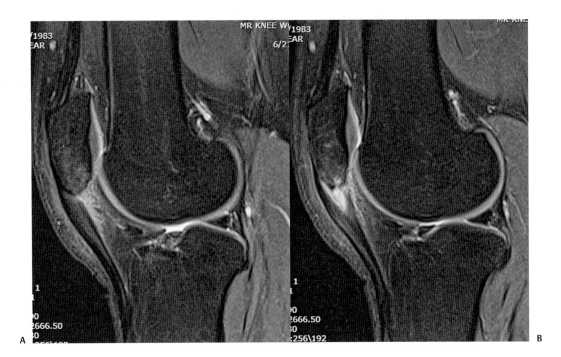

■ Clinical Presentation

A young adult athlete presents with anterior knee pain.

■ **Imaging Findings**

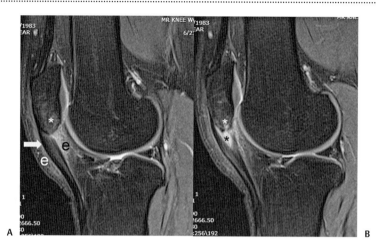

(A, B) Sagittal fluid-sensitive MR imaging of the knee shows proximal patellar tendon expansion (*arrow*) with areas of proximal interstitial tearing (*black asterisk*). There is edema (*e*) within the surrounding superficial and deep infrapatellar fat. Bone marrow edema (*white asterisk*) involves the inferior pole of the patella.

■ **Differential Diagnosis**

• ***Jumper's knee:*** An overuse injury seen within the proximal patellar tendon related to excessive jumping. Characteristic MRI findings include proximal patella tendon enlargement and interstitial tearing with surrounding soft tissue inflammation and inferior patellar marrow edema.
• *Sinding–Larsen–Johansson:* An osteochondrosis of the skeletally immature patella occurring along the distal pole at the insertion of the patellar tendon, typically sparing the patellar tendon.

■ **Essential Facts**

• Jumper's knee represents proximal patellar tendinosis.
• Injury occurs with repetitive overloading of the extensor mechanism of the knee in sports that require explosive jumping movements, such as basketball, volleyball, and soccer.
• Patients present with pain at the proximal insertion of the patellar tendon.
• This process occurs in active, skeletally mature males as mechanical stress is transferred from the patella to the tissues of the proximal patellar tendon.
• Tendinopathy typically involves the proximal and medial one third of the patellar tendon which exhibits T2 signal increase on MRI.
• The proximal patellar tendon exhibits swelling and enlargement beyond the normal anterior posterior thickness of 7 mm.
• Additional MRI features include surrounding soft tissue edema/inflammation with or without marrow edema of the inferior patellar pole.

■ **Other Imaging Findings**

• Focal soft tissue swelling and fullness adjacent to the inferior pole of the patella may be observed on lateral knee radiographs.
• Ultrasound imaging demonstrates a swollen, hypoechoic proximal patellar tendon.

✓ **Pearls and ✗ Pitfalls**

✓ Chronic jumper's knee may cause protuberant bone formation along the inferior pole of the patella, resulting in an elongated patella on lateral knee radiographs.
✗ Sagittal fluid-sensitive MR images frequently show minimal normal signal increase within the proximal posterior patellar tendon at the patellar insertion.

Case 69

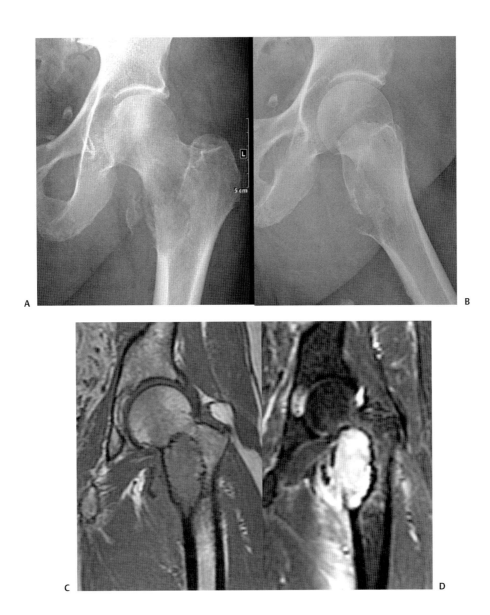

■ Clinical Presentation

A 75-year-old patient presents with atraumatic acute worsening of left hip pain.

■ Imaging Findings

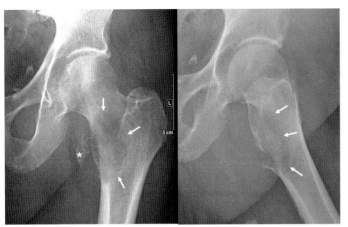
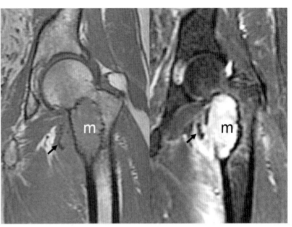

A, B   C, D

(A, B) Radiographs of the left hip demonstrate a medially displaced avulsion fracture (*asterisk*) of the left lesser trochanter. Ill-defined corticomedullary lytic changes (*arrows*) are seen at the harvest site of the avulsion fracture. **(C, D)** Coronal fat-sensitive and fluid-sensitive MR images through the left hip demonstrate a geographic intramedullary mass (*m*) exhibiting intermediate T1 and hyperintense T2 signal with surrounding soft tissue and bone marrow edema. The medially displaced low signal lesser trochanteric cortical avulsion fracture fragment (*arrow*) is surrounded by fluid/edema.

■ Differential Diagnosis

• **Pathologic fracture (lesser trochanter avulsion):** An atraumatic avulsion fracture of the lesser trochanter superimposed upon lytic bony changes from a metastasis. MRI findings of a geographic intramedullary lesion at the level of the fracture bed exhibiting intermediate to diminished T1 and hyperintense T2 signal further support this diagnosis.

■ Essential Facts

• Avulsion fractures of the lesser trochanter result from traction applied by the iliopsoas muscle and tendon.
• This is a rare traumatic injury seen in the young athlete.
• An adult presenting with this particular avulsion fracture, particularly an older adult without a history of trauma, has high likelihood of having an underlying malignancy.
• The most common lesion is a metastasis.
• Radiographs may demonstrate aggressive lytic bony changes at the site of the fracture, enabling an appropriate diagnosis.
• MRI is recommended for further characterization of these lesions.
• Typical MR features of an underlying bone marrow malignancy include a geographic region of bone marrow replacement displaying intermediate to hypointense T1 signal with corresponding T2 signal hyperintensity.

■ Other Imaging Findings

• CT findings of a pathologic fracture include periosteal reaction with cortical and trabecular destruction.

✓ Pearls and ✗ Pitfalls

✓ Profound T1 signal alteration on MR imaging is more sensitive and specific than T2 signal changes in discriminating between pathologic and nonpathologic fractures.
✗ Radiography often fails to display the underlying osseous lesion at the time of initial clinical presentation.

Case 70

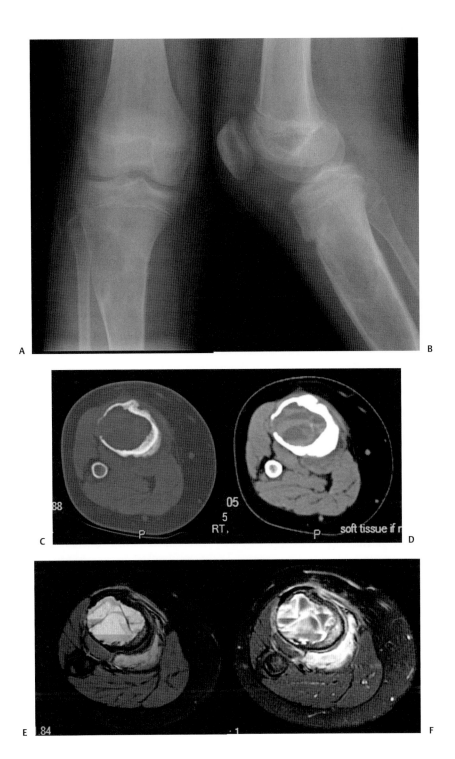

■ Clinical Presentation

A 14-year-old patient presents with leg pain.

■ **Imaging Findings**

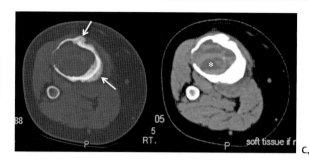

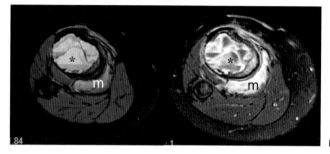

C, D

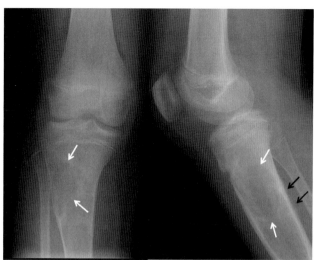

A, B

E, F

(A, B) Radiographs of the knee show a proximal tibial metadiaphyseal lytic lesion with ill-defined borders (*white arrows*) and posterior tibial periosteal reaction (*black arrows*). **(C, D)** Axial CT scan images with bone and soft tissue windows demonstrate extensive periosteal reaction (*white arrows*) with an intramedullary mass demonstrating fluid–fluid levels (*asterisk*). There is permeative cortical destruction along the lateral tibial cortex. No osteoid mineralization is seen. **(E, F)** Axial fluid-sensitive and post-gadolinium fat-suppressed MR images display marrow replacement by heterogeneous tissue with areas of high signal intensity and fluid–fluid levels (*asterisk*) demonstrating rim enhancement. There is an associated soft tissue mass (*m*) posteriorly exhibiting hyperintense T2 signal with avid enhancement.

■ **Differential Diagnosis**

- ***Telangiectatic osteosarcoma:*** A variant of osteosarcoma resulting in a permeative osteolytic lesion without appreciable osteoid matrix with superimposed fluid–fluid levels and an associated soft tissue mass.
- *Aneurysmal bone cyst:* A benign circumscribed lucent metaphyseal lesion without periostitis containing fluid–fluid levels on CT and MRI. This lesion does not contain a soft tissue mass and presents in the first or second decade of life.
- *Giant cell tumor:* An eccentric, circumscribed, and expansile epiphyseal lesion containing internal bony septations seen in the adult skeleton, not typically accompanied by a soft tissue mass, is consistent with this tumor.

■ **Essential Facts**

- Telangiectatic osteosarcoma represents 12% of all osteosarcomas.
- This lesion has a predilection for the long bones, most notably the distal femur.

- These patients may present with pain and swelling, with or without pathologic fractures.
- Radiographs and CT imaging demonstrate osteolysis without significant bone formation.
- Central hemorrhagic locules account for the fluid–fluid levels seen on CT and MRI.
- These aneurysmally dilated cavities contain blood with superimposed high-grade sarcomatous cells along the intervening septations.

■ **Other Imaging Findings**

- Radionuclide bone scan demonstrates the "doughnut sign" represented by peripheral radiotracer uptake in the solid portion of the lesion with central photopenia secondary to the hemorrhagic locules.

✓ **Pearls and ✗ Pitfalls**

✓ A soft tissue mass frequently coexists with this lesion.

✗ A traumatized aneurysmal bone cyst may share similar features with telangiectatic osteosarcoma.

Case 71

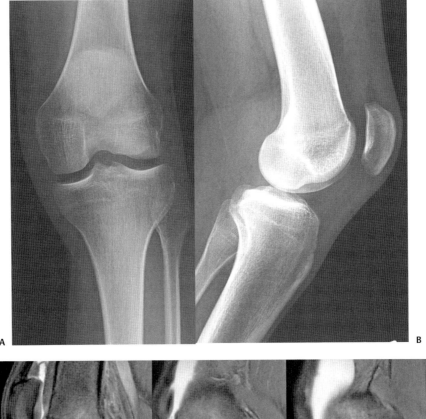

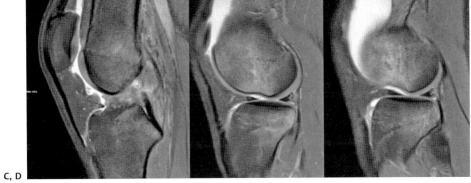

■ Clinical Presentation

A patient presents with a twisting injury with knee pain and swelling.

■ Imaging Findings

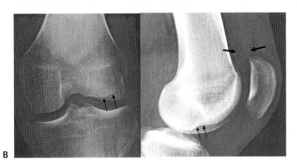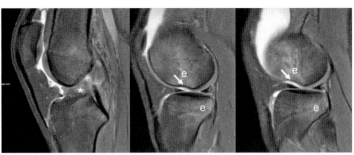

A, B   C, D, E

(A, B) Radiographs of the knee show an abnormally deep depression over the lateral condylopatellar sulcus (*thin black arrows*). A large joint effusion (*thick black arrows*) is also present. **(C–E)** Sagittal fluid-sensitive MR images show complete disruption of the anterior cruciate ligament (ACL; *asterisk*). An osteochondral depression (*white arrow*) is located anteriorly along the lateral femoral condyle, accounting for the deepening of the lateral condylopatellar sulcus. Edematous contusions (*e*) involve the lateral condyle and posterior lateral tibial plateau.

■ Differential Diagnosis

• ***Anterior cruciate ligament tear (deep sulcus sign):***
A deepened lateral condylopatellar sulcus, or lateral femoral notch sign, results from impaction injury by the posterior margin of the lateral tibial plateau related to rupture of the ACL. The lateral femoral condyle and lateral tibial plateau edema on MRI represent kissing contusions as a result of this injury. MRI findings of ACL disruption confirm the diagnosis.

■ Essential Facts

• ACL injuries occur with a valgus load to the knee in various states of flexion with external rotation of the tibia or internal rotation of the femur.
• This type of injury usually occurs with maneuvers such as rapid deceleration and simultaneous directional change termed pivot shift.
• These maneuvers stress the ACL and result in rupture, allowing anterior subluxation of the tibia relative to the femur.

• Disruption of the ACL most commonly occurs in the midsubstance.
• Impaction of the lateral femoral condyle against the posterolateral margin of the lateral tibial plateau causes kissing bone marrow contusions on MR imaging.
• Surgical repair is required.

✓ Pearls and ✗ Pitfalls

✓ A lateral femoral condylar osteochondral depression of > 2.0 mm in depth is highly suggestive of an ACL injury and is termed the lateral femoral notch sign.
✗ A prominent normal lateral condylopatellar sulcus may exist causing confusion with the lateral femoral notch sign.
✗ The lateral femoral notch sign is not frequently encountered with ACL tears.

Case 72

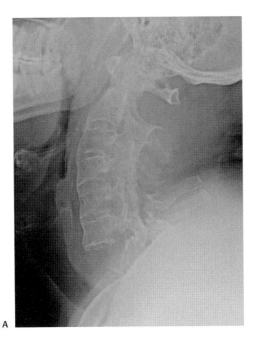

A

■ **Clinical Presentation**

A 60-year-old patient status post fall from standing presents with neurologic symptoms.

■ **Further Work-up**

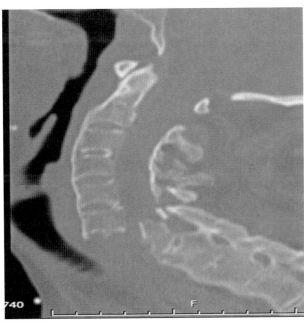

B

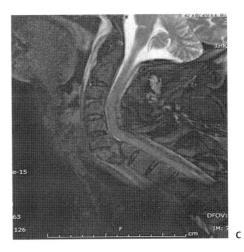

C

■ Imaging Findings

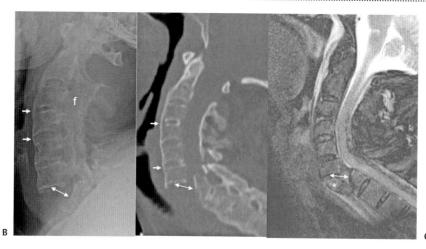

A, B   C

(A–C) Lateral radiograph of the cervical spine demonstrates smooth syndesmophyte formation (*white arrows*) adhering to and bridging successive verte-bral bodies with fusion through the facet joints (*f*). Disruption through the C6–C7 intervertebral disk space is present (*double arrow*). Sagittal reformatted CT scan demonstrates the anterior bridging vertebral body syndesmophytes (*white arrows*) and disk space disruption at C6–C7 (*double arrow*). Sagittal fluid-sensitive MR sequence through the C6–C7 disruption (*double arrow*) demonstrates a disrupted anterior longitudinal ligament replaced with a lobu-lated low-signal hematoma (*asterisk*).

■ Differential Diagnosis

• **Ankylosing spondylitis (AS):** A seronegative spondyloarthropathy causing smooth syndesmophyte formation which bridges multiple vertebral bodies with associated facet joint osseous fusion. Associated disruption through the C6–C7 intervertebral disk space in this patient with minimal trauma represents a complication of this disorder.
• *Diffuse idiopathic skeletal hyperostosis (DISH):* A degenerative process resulting in bulky paravertebral ossification which does not demonstrate smooth bridging with the underlying vertebral bodies.

■ Essential Facts

• AS represents a chronic inflammatory arthritic condition, frequently seen in young men between the ages of 15 and 35 years.
• This disease process primarily affects the axial skeleton, synovial/cartilaginous joints, and entheses.
• Erosive changes are followed by bone formation with eventual fusion, typically affecting the sacroiliac joints and spine.
• Many patients are HLA-B27 positive, suggesting a hereditary component.
• Fractures in these patients are four times more common than in the general population, related to the relatively rigid spine and kyphotic deformity.
• Spinal fractures in AS most commonly involve the cervical spine.
• Alteration of the normal spinal biomechanics occurs as a result of syndesmophyte formation with ossification of the spinal ligaments and annulus.

• These fractures are typically sustained from a low-energy mechanism, such as a fall from standing.
• Many of these fractures traverse the intervertebral disk space.
• Typical mechanism of injury is hyperextension with involvement of all three columns, resembling a seatbelt-type injury, with significant coexisting neurologic injury.
• A low threshold should exist for obtaining CT and or MR imaging in patients with AS following cervical spine trauma.

■ Other Imaging Findings

• CT imaging will display acute cortical interruption, particularly evident through the spinous processes and facets.
• MR imaging may reveal bony contusion, soft tissue swelling, longitudinal ligament disruption, and spinal cord contusion.

✓ Pearls and ✗ Pitfalls

✓ Cervical spine fractures in these patients are particularly common at C5–C6 and C6–C7 secondary to mobility of the skull and the relative rigid fixation of the adjoining thoracic spine.
✗ Radiographs may fail to display the cervical spine fractures secondary to superimposed kyphotic deformities and distorted anatomy.

Case 73

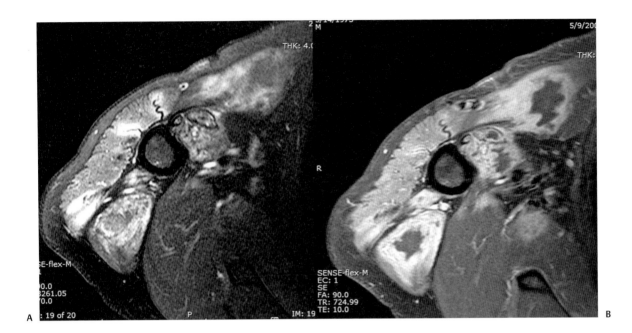

■ Clinical Presentation

A patient with a drug overdose was found face down and unconscious.

■ Imaging Findings

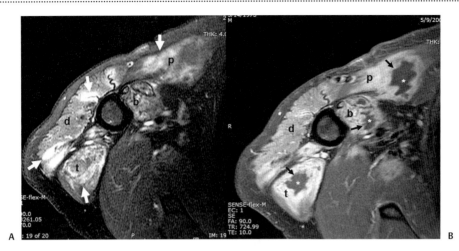

(A) Axial fluid-sensitive and **(B)** T1 fat-suppressed post-gadolinium images through the shoulder and proximal humerus demonstrate patchy intramuscular T2 signal increase (*white arrows*) within the pectoralis (*p*), deltoid (*d*), biceps brachii (*b*), and triceps (*t*) musculature. Areas of rim enhancement (*black arrows*) surrounding central nonenhancing muscle tissue (*asterisk*) are seen at the level of the pectoralis, biceps, and triceps.

■ Differential Diagnosis

- **Muscle infarct:** A condition related to diminished or absent intramuscular blood flow exhibiting MRI findings of patchy muscle edema with corresponding irregular mosaic and/or rim enhancement patterns following gadolinium administration.
- *Pyomyositis:* A disease process typically seen in immunocompromised patients with MR features of an irregular, heterogeneous intramuscular hyperintense T2 fluid collection with rim enhancement following gadolinium administration.
- *Muscle strain:* A posttraumatic process resulting in muscle fiber architectural disruption with MRI findings ranging from mild muscle edema to frank fiber disruption with interposed fluid and hematoma formation.

■ Essential Facts

- Muscle infarction, also known as *myonecrosis,* may result from localized trauma/closed fractures, thermal injury, infection, heavy exercise, or continuous extrinsic pressure applied to muscle.
- The current case represents myonecrosis secondary to persistent extrinsic pressure applied to the shoulder girdle musculature against the hard surface of the floor.
- Pathophysiology relates to increased pressure within a confined fascial space resulting in venous occlusion with subsequent ischemia and muscle infarct.

- Patients may present with exquisite tenderness to palpation of the affected compartment with neurologic symptoms associated with the affected nerves within the compartment.
- MRI findings typically consist of irregular foci of intramuscular edema on fluid-sensitive sequences with patchy irregular peripheral enhancement related to hypoperfusion.
- Early diagnosis may be achieved with utilization of a manometry probe into the affected compartment for direct pressure measurements.

■ Other Imaging Findings

- Radiographs may demonstrate sheetlike intramuscular calcific deposits secondary to chronic muscle infarction and calcific myonecrosis.

✓ Pearls and ✗ Pitfalls

- ✓ MRI findings of geographic or patchy intramuscular edema with corresponding rim enhancement or a mosaic enhancement pattern should raise suspicion for muscle infarction.
- ✗ Early MRI findings are nonspecific, showing diffuse intramuscular T2 signal increase related to increased fluid content within the musculature.

Case 74

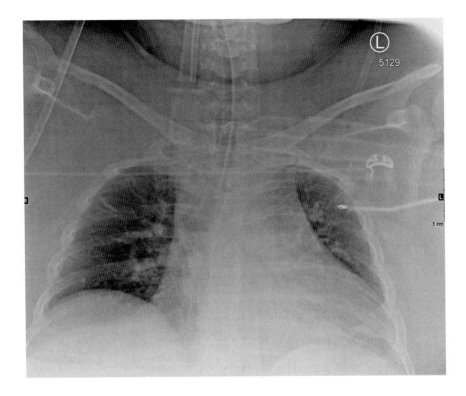

■ Clinical Presentation

A patient presents with a pulseless right upper extremity following a motor vehicle collision with ejection.

■ Imaging Findings

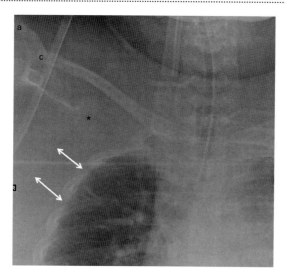

Portable frontal chest radiograph demonstrates an endotracheal tube in place. The right scapula is laterally displaced from the chest wall (*double arrows*) with disarticulation of the acromioclavicular joint, distal articular margin of the clavicle (*c*), and acromion (*a*). A displaced fracture through the medial border of the scapula (*asterisk*) is seen.

■ Differential Diagnosis

- **Scapulothoracic dissociation (STD):** A posttraumatic process affecting the shoulder girdle causing lateral scapular disarticulation from the thoracic wall.

■ Essential Facts

- STD represents an infrequent traumatic injury with potentially devastating outcomes.
- This is considered a closed forequarter amputation with complete disruption of the musculotendinous attachments to the chest wall.
- Mechanism of injury is traction force applied to the shoulder girdle as seen in motorcycle or motor vehicle collision.
- The upper extremity may be flaccid as a result of associated brachial plexus injury and/or nerve root avulsions.
- Imaging demonstrates lateral displacement of the scapula with disruption of the sternoclavicular and/or acromioclavicular joints with associated scapular and/or clavicle fractures.
- There is complete loss of the scapulothoracic articulation, with massive swelling related to hematoma formation from subclavian and/or axillary artery avulsion creating a pulseless extremity.
- Mortality rates associated with this injury are high.
- Long-term complications include ischemia and paralysis, with possible amputation required.

■ Other Imaging Findings

- CT angiogram will demonstrate interruption of contrast with or without extravasation at the level of the lateral subclavian and/or axillary artery.

✓ Pearls and ✗ Pitfalls

- ✓ A scapulothoracic ratio may be measured on axial CT imaging through the chest and represents the distance from the spinous process to a specific point on each scapula, normally ranging from 1.07 to 1.15. Any variation beyond this range should raise suspicion for STD.
- ✗ STD may be difficult to detect on radiographs with suboptimal patient positioning and portable technique.

Case 75

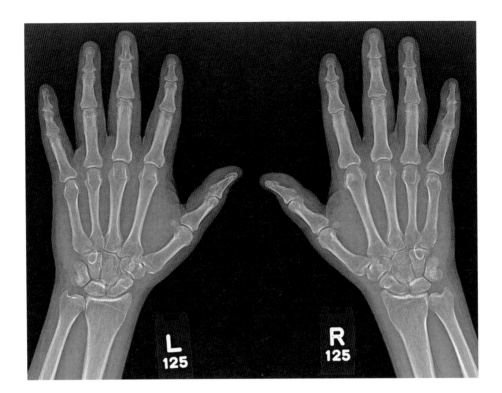

▪ Clinical Presentation

A young adult male patient presents with arthralgias.

■ **Imaging Findings**

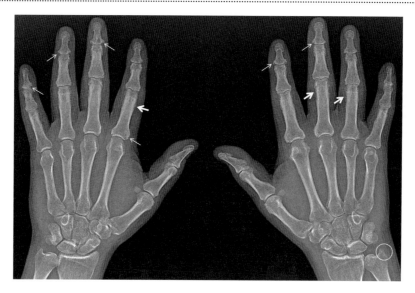

Radiographs of the bilateral hands show marginal periarticular erosions with adjacent irregular bone proliferation (*thin arrows*) in a bilateral, irregular distribution along the metacarpophalangeal (MCP), proximal interphalangeal (PIP), and distal interphalangeal (DIP) joints. Mild periosteal reaction outlines the proximal phalanges (*thick arrows*). Asymmetric ulnar styloid erosion (*encircled*) is present. No osteopenia or subluxations are seen.

■ **Differential Diagnosis**

• ***Psoriatic arthritis (PA):*** A seronegative spondyloarthropathy notable for bilateral and irregular distribution of periarticular erosions admixed with bone proliferation affecting the MCP and PIP/DIP joints, with phalangeal periosteal reaction. There is typically absence of osteopenia in psoriatic arthritis.
• *Rheumatoid arthritis:* An erosive, deforming inflammatory arthropathy composed of periarticular osteopenia with symmetric erosions centered around the MCP and PIP joints.
• *Osteoarthritis:* A degenerative condition composed of joint space narrowing, sclerosis, and marginal osteophyte formation centered at the DIP joints of the hands without erosions.

■ **Essential Facts**

• PA is a chronic, inflammatory, and proliferative disease of the skin commonly affecting Caucasians.
• Genetic, environmental, and immunologic factors have been considered to play key roles in the development and expression of PA.
• As many as 60% of patients with PA are HLA-B27 positive, with mean age at diagnosis of ~40 years.
• Skin manifestations precede the development of arthritis, which may be bilateral or unilateral, symmetric or asymmetric.

• The hands and feet are the most commonly involved locations in PA.
• Involvement of several joints in a single digit, with soft tissue swelling, produce what appears clinically as a "sausage digit."
• Erosions typically begin at the margins of the joint and erode the articular surface, progressing along the joint capsule away from the joint.
• Bone proliferation produces an irregular and indistinct appearance to the marginal bone about the involved joint, characterized as a "fuzzy" appearance or "whiskering."
• Erosive changes of the joint may take the appearance of a "pencil and cup," with one end of the joint forming a cup and the other a pencil that projects into this cup.
• Bone mineralization is typically preserved.

✓ **Pearls and ✗ Pitfalls**

✓ Bone proliferation on radiographs is one of the distinguishing features of this condition in the hands.
✓ DIP involvement is usually present in the hands.
✗ The occasional asymmetric and monoarticular distribution of PA may mimic an infectious process.

Case 76

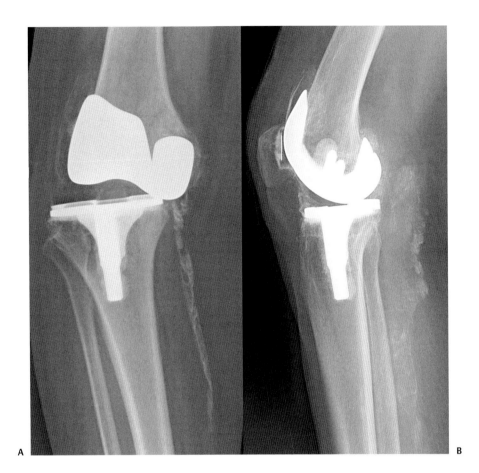

A   B

■ Clinical Presentation

A patient status post total knee arthroplasty 12 years ago presents with joint fullness and limping.

■ **Imaging Findings**

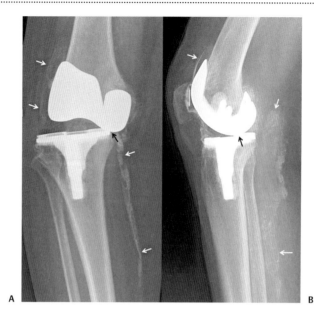

A   B

(A, B) Radiographs of the knee show total arthroplasty changes with varus angulation. Metal-on-metal contact is seen between the medial femoral con-dylar prosthesis and medial tibial tray (*black arrows*). Radiodense debris outlines the suprapatellar bursa and posterior capsule (*white arrows*), creating a "metal line sign." This line extends along the posterior and medial proximal leg along the expected course of a Baker's cyst.

■ **Differential Diagnosis**

• *Metallosis:* Metallic debris shed from arthroplasty components as a result of metal-on-metal contact. This process results in metallic opacification of the synovial capsule along with a dense effusion.

■ **Essential Facts**

• Metallosis is an uncommon and late complication of arthroplasty which occurs after failure and/or wear of the interposed polyethylene weight-bearing surfaces.
• Subsequent contact between the metal components allows abrasion and shedding of metallic fragments.
• This debris outlines the synovial lining of the joint capsule, creating a "metal line sign" on radiographs.
• A dense joint effusion may be present, appearing as black synovial fluid upon aspiration.
• Metallosis most commonly afflicts the knee.

■ **Other Imaging Findings**

• MR imaging reveals thickened synovium exhibiting low signal intensity on all pulse sequences.

✓ **Pearls and** ✗ **Pitfalls**

✓ An aggressive osteolytic response may be seen in the setting of metallosis, particularly along the acetabular component of total hip arthroplasty.
✗ A component of aseptic lymphocytic vasculitis-associated lesions may be seen within the soft tissues of patients with metallosis, complicating the diagnosis.

Case 77

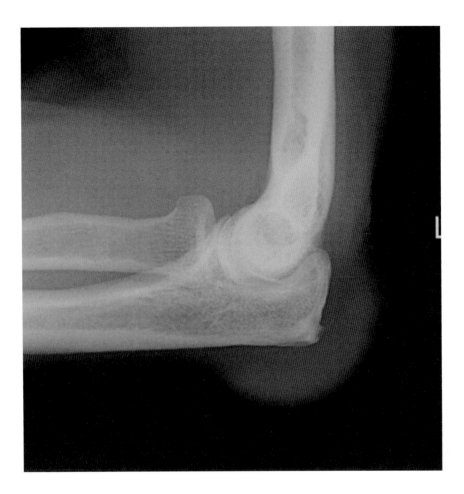

■ Clinical Presentation

A patient presents with chronic elbow fullness with mild tenderness.

■ Imaging Findings

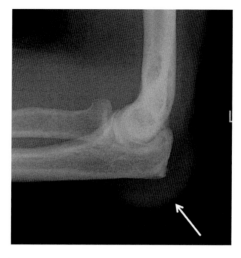

Lateral radiograph of the elbow demonstrates soft tissue fullness (*arrow*) superficial to the olecranon.

■ Differential Diagnosis

- **Olecranon bursitis:** Soft tissue fullness superficial to the olecranon on lateral radiographs of the elbow secondary to underlying inflammation, trauma, or infection are diagnostic features of this condition.
- *Ganglion cyst:* A juxta-articular or juxta-tendinous fluid-filled mass frequently seen around the hand and wrist.

■ Essential Facts

- The olecranon bursa is a subcutaneous space lined by a synovial membrane posterior to the olecranon.
- The synovial lining of the olecranon bursa secretes synovial fluid to provide smooth motion between the superficial skin surface and the olecranon.
- Causes of inflammation and fullness of the olecranon bursa include rheumatoid arthritis, gout, infection, hemorrhage, and repetitive microtrauma.
- Traumatic bursitis accounts for most cases.
- Olecranon bursitis is typically a clinical diagnosis.

■ Other Imaging Findings

- MRI of the elbow will demonstrate olecranon bursal fluid distention manifested by internal T1 signal decrease and T2 signal increase with rim enhancement. Occasionally, reactive olecranon bone marrow edema is seen.
- Ultrasound imaging will show hypoechoic fluid distention of the bursa.

✓ Pearls and ✗ Pitfalls

- ✓ Inflammation of the olecranon bursa is frequently the initial presentation of gout and most commonly occurs with recurrent episodes of gouty arthritis.
- ✗ In the absence of a clinical history and significant extrabursal soft tissue swelling, infectious bursitis may be difficult to distinguish from other noninfectious causes of bursitis.

Case 78

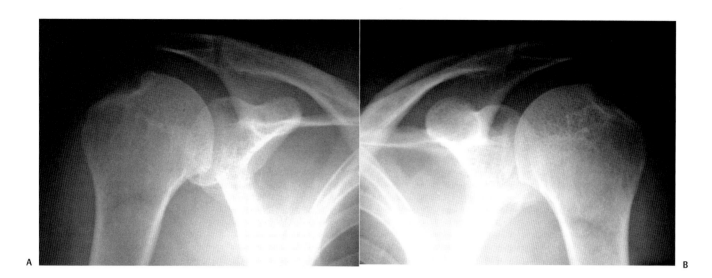

A   B

■ Clinical Presentation

A young adult male patient presents with chronic low back pain and atraumatic bilateral shoulder pain.

■ **Imaging Findings**

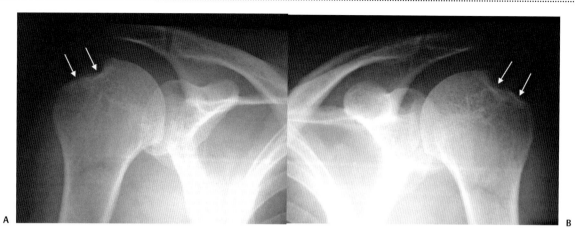

(A, B) Frontal radiographs of both shoulders demonstrate bony erosions bordered by sclerosis along the lateral proximal margins of the humeral heads (*arrows*) involving the greater tuberosities. These radiographic findings are consistent with hatchet deformities.

■ **Differential Diagnosis**

- *Ankylosing spondylitis (AS) hatchet deformities:* Normal bone mineralization with symmetric bilateral humeral head greater tuberosity erosive changes in a young adult male with low back pain are diagnostic features of this seronegative inflammatory spondyloarthropathy.
- *Rheumatoid arthritis:* A seropositive inflammatory arthropathy with signature findings in the shoulder composed of joint space loss and osteopenia with a high-riding humeral head related to rotator cuff deficiency.
- *Psoriatic arthritis:* A seronegative spondyloarthropathy causing musculoskeletal bony erosions and proliferation in an asymmetric fashion frequently coexisting with skin findings of psoriatic plaques.

■ **Essential Facts**

- AS represents an HLA-B27–positive inflammatory spondyloarthropathy.
- This is a chronic inflammatory arthritic condition typically seen in young men between the ages of 15 and 35 years.
- Although this condition typically affects the axial skeleton, peripheral joints may also be affected and include the hips, knees, and glenohumeral joints.
- Inflammatory erosive changes are followed by bone formation.
- Changes in the shoulder include bilateral greater tuberosity erosions destroying portions of the greater tuberosity at the rotator cuff tendon attachment. These changes cause the humeral head to assume the shape of a hatchet on radiographs.
- Erosions of the humeral head may also occur at the site of the synovial reflection.

■ **Other Imaging Findings**

- MR imaging may reveal bone marrow edema changes within the humeral head at the site of the erosions related to enthesitis.

✓ **Pearls and ✗ Pitfalls**

- ✓ Sacroiliac joint erosions and/or ankylosis frequently coexist in patients exhibiting hatchet deformities.
- ✗ Radiographic alteration of the humeral heads may be misinterpreted as a Hill–Sachs deformity seen with anterior shoulder dislocations.

Case 79

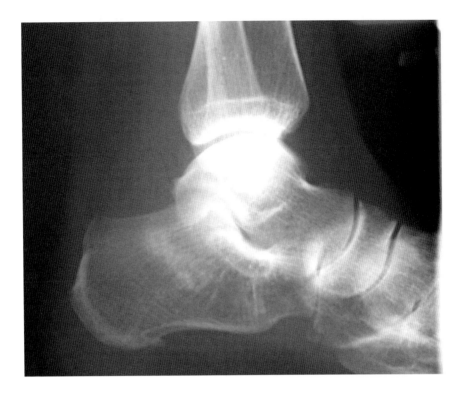

■ Clinical Presentation

An active elderly female presents with heel pain.

■ Imaging Findings

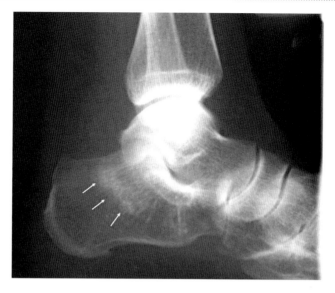

Lateral radiograph of the ankle demonstrates curvilinear sclerosis (*arrows*) through the posterior calcaneus, paralleling the posterior facet of the subtalar joint. Diffuse osteopenia is also present.

■ Differential Diagnosis

- ***Calcaneal insufficiency fracture:*** A nonacute fracture occurring on a background of osteopenia through the posterior calcaneus represented by curvilinear or irregular sclerosis on radiographs.
- *Bone island:* A focal region of compact, spiculated bone formation centered in the cortex or medullary canal, also referred to as an enostosis.
- *Bone infarct:* Focal intramedullary osteonecrosis manifesting on radiography with geographic serpentine sclerosis in a shell-like pattern.

■ Essential Facts

- Calcaneal fractures may be characterized as insufficiency fractures, fatigue/stress type fractures, or acute traumatic fractures.
- Insufficiency fractures may be seen in patients with diminished bone mineral density, such as the postmenopausal osteoporotic female, as in this case.
- Normal forces applied to this weakened bone result in these types of fractures.
- Fatigue/stress calcaneal fractures result from excessive force applied to normal bone stock.
- The opposing force of the Achilles tendon contributes to both the fatigue/stress and insufficiency type calcaneal fractures.
- These types of calcaneal fractures are typically extra-articular in location.

■ Other Imaging Findings

- Radionuclide bone scan demonstrates increased radio-tracer uptake along the fracture site.
- MRI findings consist of a linear low T1/low T2 signal intramedullary defect surrounded by marked bone marrow edema changes.

✓ Pearls and ✗ Pitfalls

- ✓ Calcaneal insufficiency fractures typically parallel the posterior facet of the subtalar joint.
- ✗ In the early stages of calcaneal insufficiency fractures, radiographs appear normal, requiring ~2 weeks after onset of pain before detection on radiographs.

Case 80

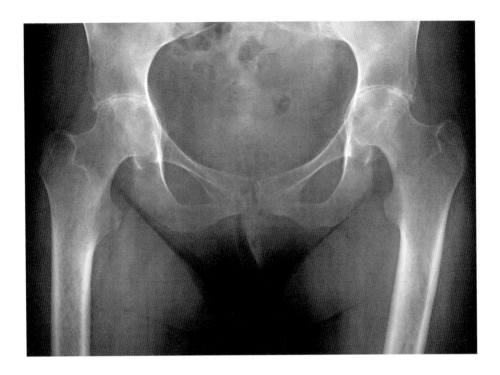

■ **Clinical Presentation**

A 55-year-old female patient presents with a history of polyarthralgias.

■ Imaging Findings

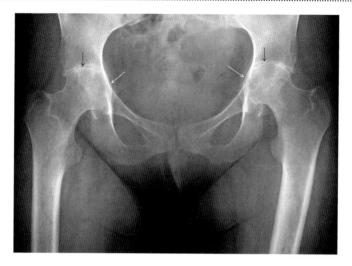

Frontal radiograph of the pelvis demonstrates diffuse osteopenia. There is uniform bilateral hip joint space loss. Medial acetabular wall protrusion (*white arrows*) is present with subchondral cortical erosive change involving the acetabula and femoral heads (*black arrows*). Osteophyte formation is minimal.

■ Differential Diagnosis

- ***Rheumatoid arthritis (RA):*** An inflammatory and erosive arthropathy characterized by osteopenia, symmetric and uniform joint space loss of the hips with medial acetabular wall protrusion, erosive changes, and paucity of osteophyte formation.
- *Osteoarthritis:* A degenerative condition characterized by superolateral femoral acetabular joint space narrowing with sclerosis and osteophytosis.
- *Septic arthritis:* A destructive, monoarticular process with radiographic findings of periarticular osteopenia, gradual joint space loss, and bony erosive changes with soft tissue swelling.

■ Essential Facts

- RA is a chronic, systemic, polyarticular disease that predominantly involves synovial joints in a symmetric fashion.
- This disease affects 0.5 to 1.0% of the global population, with females affected more frequently than males.
- Patients are typically 30 to 60 years of age.
- Rheumatoid factor antibody binds to antigens within the synovial membranes, causing local inflammatory changes with synovial thickening.
- The radiographic findings of RA are typically symmetric and include osteopenia, soft tissue swelling, periarticular erosions, and joint space loss.

- Hip involvement in RA tends to occur later in the disease process.
- Characteristic radiographic findings in the hips include bilateral and concentric femoral acetabular joint space loss with medial acetabular protrusion, and erosive changes along the femoral head and acetabular subchondral bone plate.

■ Other Imaging Findings

- MR imaging of active RA demonstrates synovial thickening and a joint effusion manifested by soft tissue fullness with intermediate T2 signal increase distending the joint capsule.
- Ultrasound imaging of a joint with active RA demonstrates abnormal, hypoechoic, intra-articular soft tissue fullness with increased color Doppler flow.

✓ Pearls and ✗ Pitfalls

✓ A young female patient demonstrating osteopenia with symmetric uniform narrowing of the hips should raise suspicion for RA.

✗ Synovial thickening and fluid distention of the iliopsoas bursa may extend into the inguinal and lower pelvic soft tissues, masquerading as a cystic mass on cross-sectional imaging.

✗ An accurate diagnosis of end-stage RA may be compromised by the development of secondary osteoarthritis.

Case 81

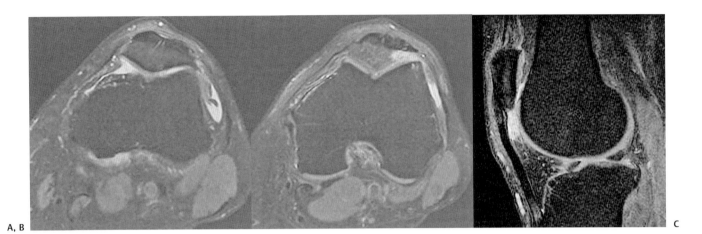

A, B   C

■ Clinical Presentation

A 42-year-old female patient presents with chronic lateral knee pain and instability.

■ **Imaging Findings**

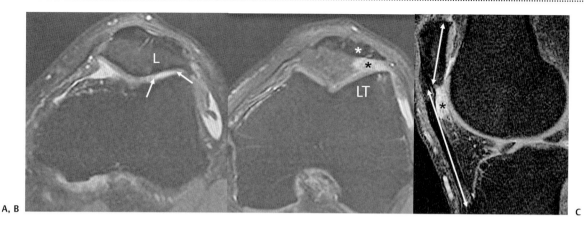

A, B

C

(A, B) Axial fat-sensitive MR images through the knee display increased signal (*black asterisk*) within the lateral aspect of Hoffa's fat pad between the lateral patellar tendon and lateral trochlear ridge (*LT*). The lateral margin of the patellar tendon (*white asterisk*) approximates the lateral trochlear ridge. Full-thickness chondral loss (*short arrows*) is seen along the lateral patellar facet (*L*). **(C)** Sagittal fluid-sensitive MR image re-demonstrates lateral Hoffa's fat pad edema (*black asterisk*). The length of the patellar tendon is >1.3 times the maximal patellar height (*double arrows*) representative of patella alta.

■ **Differential Diagnosis**

• ***Patellofemoral maltracking with fat pad impingement:***
Abnormal lateral patellofemoral tracking occurring with knee flexion and extension.

■ **Essential Facts**

• Patellofemoral maltracking with associated fat pad impingement represents an abnormality of patellofemoral biomechanics.
• This condition is typically seen in young, active adults, related to acute trauma or chronic repetitive stress.
• Patellar malalignment results in frictional changes between the lateral trochlear ridge, the lateral margin of Hoffa's fat, and the patellar tendon.
• MRI is reliable in identifying risk factors for chronic patellar instability.
• Patella alta is frequently present in this condition, resulting in patellar maltracking with eventual high-grade lateral patellar facet chondral loss.

• Patella alta may be measured on sagittal MR images and is present when the length of the patellar tendon exceeds 1.3 times the longest superior inferior height of the patella.
• A lateralized tibial tuberosity is seen with this condition, contributing to patellofemoral malalignment and maltracking.
• Edema will be localized to the superior and lateral aspect of Hoffa's fat on MR imaging.

✓ **Pearls and** ✗ **Pitfalls**

✓ Focal lateral proximal patellar tendinopathy is seen adjacent to the lateral trochlear ridge secondary to abnormal bony contact at this site.
✗ Static MR images fail to directly confirm the dynamic impingement related to the patellar malalignment.
✗ Superior lateral hoffitis may be seen in asymptomatic patients.

Case 82

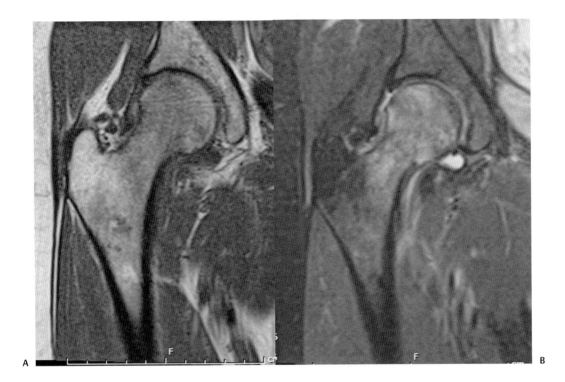

■ Clinical Presentation

A pregnant young adult patient presents with a 2-week history of atraumatic right hip pain.

■ Imaging Findings

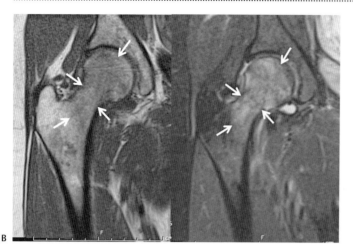
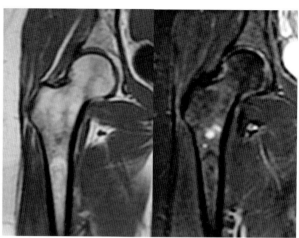

A, B　　C, D

(A, B) Coronal fat-sensitive and fluid-sensitive MR images through the right hip demonstrate diffusely diminished T1 signal and increased T2 signal (*arrows*) extending throughout the femoral head and neck. A small joint effusion is present. Joint spaces are maintained and no erosions are seen. **(C, D)** Coronal fat-sensitive and fluid-sensitive MR images through the right hip 6 months later following symptom resolution demonstrate reestablishment of normal marrow signal intensity throughout the femoral head and neck.

■ Differential Diagnosis

- **Transient bone marrow edema:** A self-limiting and idiopathic process causing bone marrow edema changes on MRI which are isolated to the femoral head and neck without joint space loss, erosions, or synovial thickening.
- **Septic arthritis:** A monoarticular infectious process causing synovial thickening, chondral and bony erosions with subcortical intramedullary bone marrow edema, and joint space loss.
- **Stress fracture:** An overuse injury with MRI findings of bone marrow edema centered around the femoral neck cortex with or without a transversely oriented hypointense T1/T2 fracture line.

■ Essential Facts

- Transient bone marrow edema represents an idiopathic, transient, and self-limited process.
- The most commonly affected joints include the hip, knee, and ankle.
- This diagnosis was initially described in women in the 3rd trimester of pregnancy. However, it is typically seen in middle-aged men, slightly more common about the left hip.
- Patients present with disabling and acute hip pain without a history of trauma.
- Symptoms may last 6 to 8 months with recurrence or migration to the opposite hip.
- Laboratory blood values are normal.
- Radiographs demonstrate osteopenia.

- MR imaging may show changes within the first 48 hours after symptoms.
- Typical MR findings include decreased T1 and increased T2 signal within the femoral head and neck.
- A joint effusion is typical without erosions, joint space loss, or synovial thickening.
- Post-gadolinium MR imaging typically demonstrates marked enhancement of the affected bone.
- Typical treatment is with nonsteroidal anti-inflammatory drugs and protected weight bearing.

■ Other Imaging Findings

- Nuclear medicine bone scan shows radionuclide uptake in the affected joint before radiographic findings are evident.

✓ Pearls and ✗ Pitfalls

- ✓ Bone marrow edema changes involve the femoral head and neck terminating at the level of the capsular insertion on the femoral neck.
- ✗ Radiographs may be normal the first 3 to 6 weeks following symptoms and may require nearly 2 years to normalize.
- ✗ Hip aspiration may be necessary to differentiate this process from an early septic arthritis.

Case 83

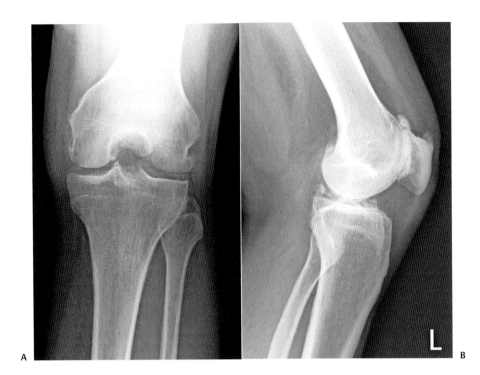

A   B

■ Clinical Presentation

An elderly male patient presents with intermittent arthralgias.

■ Imaging Findings

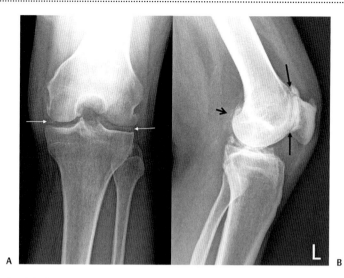

(A) Frontal and **(B)** lateral radiographs of the knee show linear calcifications within the menisci (*white arrows*) representing meniscal chondrocalcinosis. Predominantly patellofemoral osteoarthritis is seen (*long black arrows*). There is calcification involving the origin of the gastrocnemius tendons (*short black arrow*).

■ Differential Diagnosis

- ***Calcium pyrophosphate crystal deposition disease (CPPD) arthropathy:*** A crystalline-driven arthritis that frequently affects the knee joint.
- *Osteoarthritis:* A degenerative arthropathy of the knees with typical radiographic findings of marked medial femoral tibial compartment joint space loss, subchondral sclerosis, and osteophyte formation.
- *Hyperparathyroidism:* A metabolic condition causing extensive meniscal and capsular calcifications, metastatic soft tissue/vascular calcifications and bony resorptive changes.

■ Essential Facts

- CPPD arthropathy represents a crystalline-driven arthropathy frequently seen in elderly patients with an average age at presentation of 72 years.
- This disease is also referred to as *pseudogout*.
- The majority of patients are asymptomatic. However, when symptomatic, patients have a symmetric osteoarthritic-type pain.

- This arthropathy most commonly afflicts the knee joints.
- Radiographs reveal preferential joint space narrowing, sclerosis, and osteophyte formation of the patellofemoral compartment, with severe cases resulting in extrinsic scalloping of the anterior distal femoral cortex.
- Articular and periarticular crystal deposits are seen about the knee in the form of meniscal chondrocalcinosis and gastrocnemius tendon deposition.
- Treatment is aimed at symptom relief.

✓ Pearls and ✗ Pitfalls

- ✓ Lateral meniscal chondrocalcinosis and gastrocnemius tendon crystalline deposits with patellofemoral arthropathy are synonymous with this disorder.
- ✗ Many disease processes may cause secondary asymptomatic chondrocalcinosis.
- ✗ Meniscal chondrocalcinosis may mimic a meniscal tear on MRI.
- ✗ CPPD arthropathy may occur in the absence of radiographically detectable calcific deposits.

Case 84

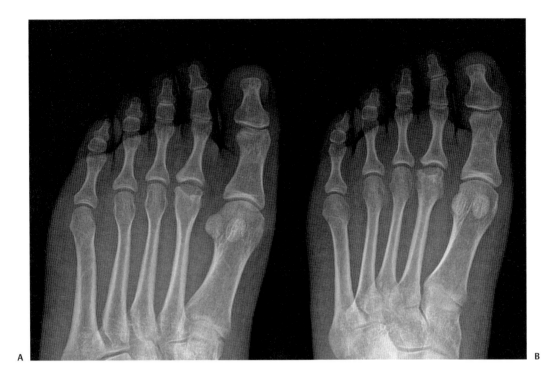

■ Clinical Presentation

A 20-year-old dancer presents with progressive forefoot pain.

■ **Imaging Findings**

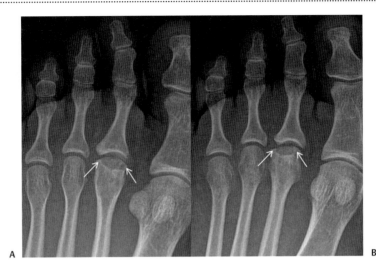

A   B

(A, B) Radiographs of the foot demonstrate geographic and circumscribed lucent bony changes (*arrows*) bordered by sclerosis along the articular surface of the second metatarsal head. Mild broadening/remodeling of this metatarsal head is seen.

■ **Differential Diagnosis**

- ***Freiberg's infraction:*** Focal osteonecrosis of the second metatarsal head.

■ **Essential Facts**

- Freiberg's infraction represents osteonecrosis of the metatarsal head.
- The pathophysiology likely relates to repetitive trauma and vascular compromise with subsequent osteochondral fracture through the distal articular surface of the metatarsal.
- The second and third metatarsals are the most commonly affected bones.
- This disorder is classically described in 12- to 18-year-old girls involved with dance and ballet presenting with focal pain and tenderness.
- High-heeled shoes have been implicated as a causative factor in older females.
- Early radiographic findings may demonstrate widening of the metatarsophalangeal joint related to an effusion.
- Radiographic findings include subchondral lucent bony changes within the metatarsal head, progressing to articular flattening, and sclerosis with eventual secondary osteoarthritic change.
- This disease process may be bilateral in up to 10% of patients.

■ **Other Imaging Findings**

- Early MR imaging demonstrates low T1 and high T2 signal intensity changes within the metatarsal head indicative of marrow edema. More advanced MRI changes may demonstrate a subchondral fracture and articular flattening with eventual decreased T1/T2 change consistent with sclerosis.

✓ **Pearls and ✗ Pitfalls**

✓ Osteoarthrosis isolated to the second or third metatarsophalangeal joint is a likely sequela of this disease.
✗ Radiographs of the foot are often negative early in the disease process.

Case 85

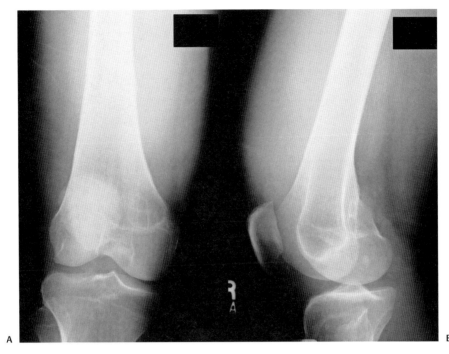

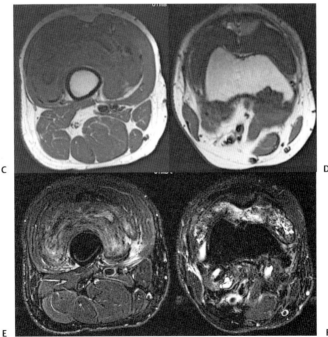

■ Clinical Presentation

A 43-year-old patient presents with knee pain and diffuse swelling.

■ Imaging Findings

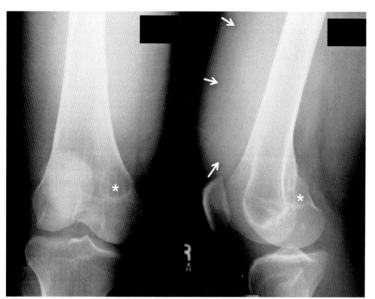

A, B

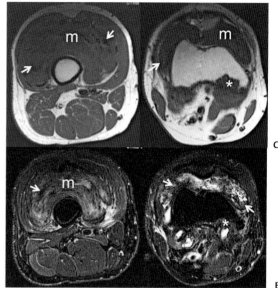

C, D

E, F

(A, B) Frontal and lateral knee radiographs show marked soft tissue swelling within the suprapatellar bursa (*arrows*) with erosive change along the posterior medial supracondylar femur (*asterisks*). There is preservation of joint spaces with normal bone density. **(C–F)** Axial fat-sensitive and fluid-sensitive MR images through the knee joint demonstrate an intermediate to low T1/T2 signal intensity intracapsular soft tissue mass (*m*). Persistent T1/T2 signal dropout (*arrows*) is seen throughout the mass. Extrinsic bony erosive changes (*asterisks*) are present at the level of the distal femur.

■ Differential Diagnosis

• ***Pigmented villonodular synovitis (PVNS):*** A monoarticular, synovial based proliferative process causing extrinsic subchondral bony erosions on radiographs. Preservation of joint spaces, absence of osteopenia combined with persistent low MR signal within a thickened synovium are characteristic features of this diagnosis.
• *Inflammatory arthropathy:* An autoimmune arthropathy represented by joint space loss with osteopenia on radiography. MRI reveals synovial thickening demonstrating intermediate to increased MR signal intensity.
• *Septic arthritis:* A monoarticular infectious arthropathy characterized by periarticular osteopenia with rapid joint space loss on radiography. MRI reveals synovial thickening exhibiting heterogeneously increased T2 signal intensity.

■ Essential Facts

• PVNS is an uncommon monoarticular disorder seen in young adults between the 3rd and 4th decades of life.
• Patients present with swelling, stiffness, and pain.
• A bloody effusion is typical.
• The knee is the most frequently involved joint, followed by the hip, ankle, and shoulder.

• This is a benign process with diffuse frondlike proliferation of synovial tissue with intracellular macrophage deposition of hemosiderin accounting for the low T1/T2 MR signal characteristics.
• Local recurrence following surgical or arthroscopic synovectomy occurs in almost 50% of cases.

■ Other Imaging Findings

• CT imaging of PVNS demonstrates diffuse synovial thickening with increased attenuation relative to muscle related to hemosiderin.

✓ Pearls and ✗ Pitfalls

✓ Calcifications on radiography exclude this diagnosis.
✗ Radiography may be normal in up to 20% of cases of PVNS.

Case 86

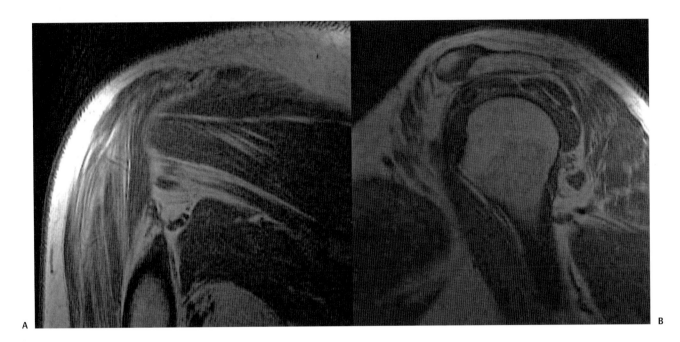

A   B

■ Clinical Presentation

A 48-year-old female patient presents with chronic shoulder pain and weakness with possible rotator cuff tear.

■ **Imaging Findings**

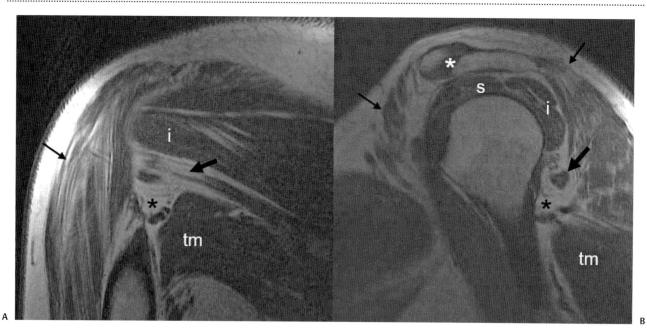

(A, B) Coronal fat-sensitive MR image through the posterior shoulder at the level of the quadrilateral space (*black asterisk*) and sagittal fat-sensitive MR image at the level of the acromioclavicular joint (*white asterisk*) demonstrate select fatty infiltration and atrophy of the deltoid (*thin black arrow*) and teres minor (*thick black arrow*). The supraspinatus (*s*), infraspinatus (*i*), and teres major (*tm*) muscles demonstrate normal size and signal intensity.

■ **Differential Diagnosis**

- *Quadrilateral space syndrome:* An entrapment neuropathy along the posterior aspect of the shoulder implicating the axillary nerve at the level of the quadrilateral space.
- *Suprascapular notch entrapment neuropathy:* A diagnosis represented by atrophy and/or edema affecting the supraspinatus and infraspinatus muscles secondary to entrapment of the suprascapular nerve at the suprascapular notch.
- *Spinoglenoid notch entrapment neuropathy:* This diagnosis is represented by atrophy and/or edema affecting the infraspinatus muscle from entrapment of the suprascapular nerve at the spinoglenoid notch.

■ **Essential Facts**

- Quadrilateral space syndrome is a potentially reversible clinical syndrome resulting from compression of the axillary nerve in the quadrilateral space.
- The axillary nerve and the posterior humeral circumflex artery traverse the quadrilateral space.
- The axillary nerve originates from the C5 and C6 neural divisions of the posterior cord of the brachial plexus and innervates the deltoid and teres minor muscles.

- The clinical manifestations include poorly localized shoulder pain, paresthesias in the affected extremity, and discrete point tenderness in the lateral aspect of the quadrilateral space.
- The typical patient is a young athlete between the ages of 25 and 35 with repetitive overhead movement of the shoulder.
- Development of fibrotic bands within the quadrilateral space impinge upon the axillary nerve.
- Resultant denervation and atrophy may affect the teres minor muscle with or without involvement of the deltoid muscle.
- MRI features include denervation edema within the musculature and loss of muscle volume with fatty infiltration.
- Muscle edema is best displayed on fluid-sensitive, fat-suppressed T2-weighted sequences, whereas fatty infiltration is best displayed on fat-sensitive T1-weighted sequences.
- Surgery is usually reserved for patients who are refractory to aggressive physical therapy.

✓ **Pearls and ✗ Pitfalls**

- ✓ Sagittal MR sequences through the mid-scapula represent the ideal imaging plane for detection of teres minor muscle changes.
- ✗ MR imaging frequently fails to display any structural abnormality responsible for this nerve impingement.

Case 87

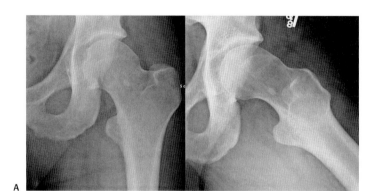

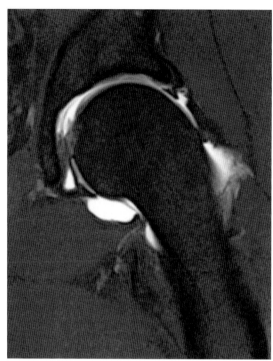

■ Clinical Presentation

A 30-year-old female patient presents with hip and groin pain.

■ Imaging Findings

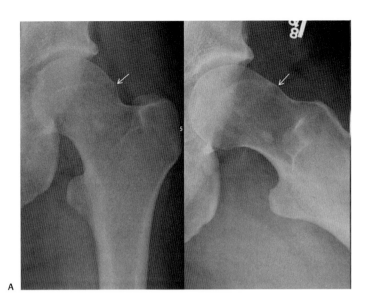 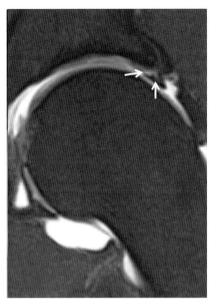

(A) Radiographs of the left hip show an aspherical contour abnormality at the superior femoral head–neck junction (*white arrows*). **(B)** Coronal T1 fat-saturated MR arthrogram of the hip demonstrates contrast extending transversely through the base of the labrum with an additional region of vertically oriented labral contrast imbibition (*white arrows*).

■ Differential Diagnosis

• **Femoral acetabular impingement (FAI) with cam deformity and labral tear:** An internal impingement disorder of the hip joint represented by an abnormal convex contour abnormality along the superior femoral head–neck junction, resulting in labral tearing.

■ Essential Facts

• FAI is characterized by pathologic, premature bony contact during hip joint motion between skeletal prominences involving the femur and/or acetabulum.
• Patients may present in the second through fourth decades of life with restricted range of motion, particularly upon flexion and internal rotation.
• Two types of FAI exist: pincer and cam type. Pincer impingement is related to overcoverage of the femoral head by the acetabulum, which is readily evident on radiographs. The cam type, as in this case, is related to an aspherical portion of the femoral head–neck junction which jams into the superior acetabulum. Radiographically, this appears as loss of the normal sphericity at the superior femoral head–neck junction. This appearance has been described as a cam deformity because the abnormal femoral bony profile resembles the appearance of a cam-type disk used in machinery.
• Most patients will have a combination of both forms of bony impingement.
• Secondary MR imaging features of this condition include superior acetabular labral tears as a result of the irregular bony contact.

• Other radiographic findings may include synovial invagination pits represented by subcentimeter lucent cystic foci along the superior margin of the femoral head–neck junction. This finding is seen as a hyperintense T2 subcortical cyst on MRI.
• Clinical signs and symptoms are essential for establishing the diagnosis of FAI, because imaging findings alone are not sufficient.
• FAI is often bilateral.
• Surgical intervention may provide immediate pain relief and entails focal osteochondroplasty at the level of the cam deformity along with repair of any labral tearing.

✓ Pearls and ✗ Pitfalls

✓ The α angle represents the most widely used measurement for assessing femoral acetabular impingement related to a cam deformity. This angle is measured on the axial view through the femoral head–neck junction and represents the angular degree at which the spherical femoral head contour becomes deformed. An abnormal measurement is > 55 degrees.
✗ Suboptimal or faulty radiographic technique of the pelvis and hip joint may over- or underestimate femoroacetabular impingement.
✗ Imaging features consistent with femoral acetabular impingement of both cam and pincer deformities are common in healthy asymptomatic male patients.

Case 88

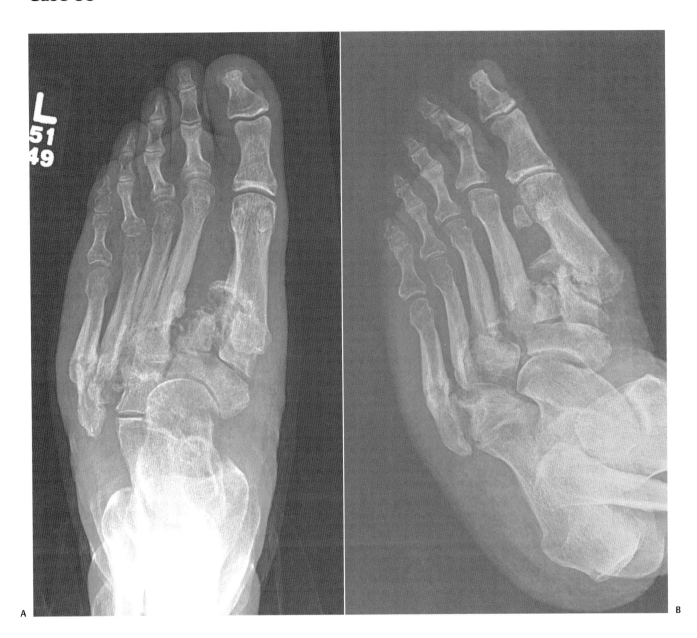

A   B

■ Clinical Presentation

A patient with chronic diabetes presents with foot deformity and diffuse swelling.

■ Imaging Findings

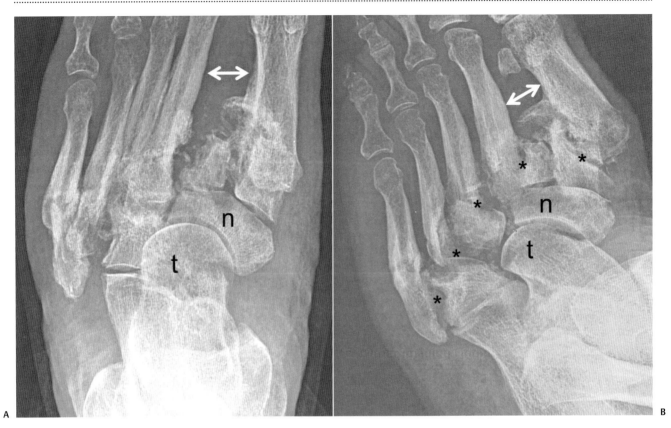

A   B

(A, B) Foot radiographs reveal extensive cortical fragmentation/osseous debris, sclerosis, disorganization, and osseous remodeling deforming the bony margins of the tarsometatarsal (TMT) joints (*asterisks*). There is widening of the first intermetatarsal space (*double arrow*) with divergent subluxation across the Lisfranc joint. Preservation of the bony architecture of the talus (*t*) and navicular (*n*) is seen with medial subluxation across this articulation. Diffuse soft tissue swelling is present.

■ Differential Diagnosis

- **Charcot arthropathy:** A neuropathic osteoarthropathy commonly seen in the diabetic foot causing extensive bony destruction with osseous debris, joint dislocation, and disorganization.
- *Osteoarthritis (OA):* A degenerative process composed of joint space loss with sclerosis and marginal osteophyte formation, typically centered at the first metatarsophalangeal joint.

■ Essential Facts

- Charcot arthropathy represents a neuropathic process secondary to an insensate joint.
- Long-standing diabetes is the most common etiology of the Charcot foot.
- Patients initially present with swelling, warmth, and erythema.
- Typical radiographic findings include joint-centered osseous destruction, dislocation/subluxation, and bony debris. These arthropathic changes are frequently centered at the TMT joints.

■ Other Imaging Findings

- MRI demonstrates a joint-centered destructive process with decreased T1 and increased T2 subcortical bone marrow signal alteration along the affected joints.

✓ Pearls and ✗ Pitfalls

- ✓ An atraumatic Lisfranc fracture/subluxation combined with radiographic findings of pedal vascular calcifications is most consistent with Charcot arthropathy secondary to diabetes.
- ✗ The bony destructive pattern of Charcot arthropathy may obscure underlying osteomyelitis in the diabetic foot.

Case 89

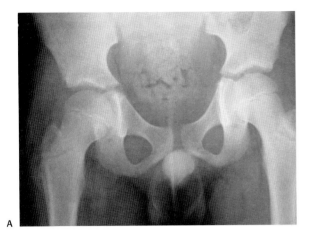

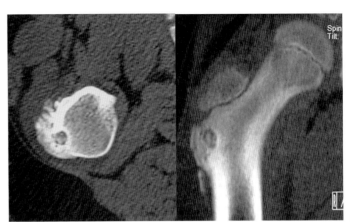

A

B, C

■ Clinical Presentation

A 9-year-old male patient presents with several weeks' history of dull, aching pain of the right hip, worse at night, with pain relief from oral nonsteroidal anti-inflammatory drugs (NSAIDs).

■ Imaging Findings

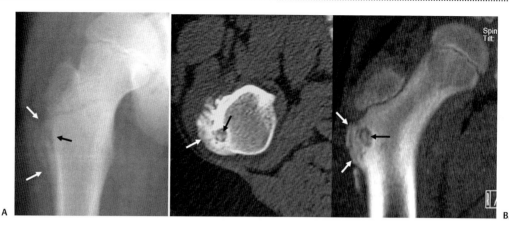

(A) Frontal view of the right hip demonstrates a segment of fusiform cortical thickening and periosteal reaction (*white arrows*) encircling a faint lucency (*black arrow*) at the level of the proximal lateral femoral cortex. **(B)** Axial and **(C)** coronal reformatted CT images show a calcified intracortical nidus (*black arrows*) embedded within the lateral femoral cortical thickening and periosteal reaction (*white arrows*).

■ Differential Diagnosis

- **Osteoid osteoma:** A cortical-based benign lesion causing fusiform cortical thickening with a calcified nidus causing symptoms of nocturnal pain relieved by NSAIDs.
- *Brodie's abscess:* A cortical medullary-based abscess manifesting radiographically as a focal lucency with irregular periosteal reaction. A sinus tract through the cortex may be present along with signs and symptoms of infection.
- *Stress fracture:* An overuse injury demonstrating periosteal reaction, cortical thickening, or a transversely oriented unicortical fracture involving major weight-bearing long bones.

■ Essential Facts

- Osteoid osteoma is a nonmalignant, vascular, and osteoblastic neoplasm.
- This lesion may be cortical, medullary, or subperiosteal in location, with the majority localized to the cortex of the tibia and femur, measuring up to 1.5 cm in size.
- This tumor represents ~12% of all benign skeletal lesions and is commonly seen in young white males.
- Patients typically present with night pain relieved by NSAIDs.
- Typical radiographic findings include an intracortical, lucent nidus with or without a central calcification with surrounding fusiform cortical thickening involving a single cortex.
- CT imaging is the modality of choice for characterization and localization of the nidus.
- Patients may be successfully treated with radio-frequency thermal ablation, although spontaneous regression may occasionally occur over time, particularly in patients treated with NSAIDs.

■ Other Imaging Findings

- Radionuclide bone scan may show the "double density sign" composed of a central focus of extremely high isotope uptake surrounded by less intense uptake related to milder bony remodeling.

✓ Pearls and ✕ Pitfalls

- ✓ The majority of femoral osteoid osteomas are proximal in location within the intertrochanteric femur or hip joint capsule.
- ✕ Extensive cortical periosteal remodeling may prevent nidus identification on radiography.

Case 90

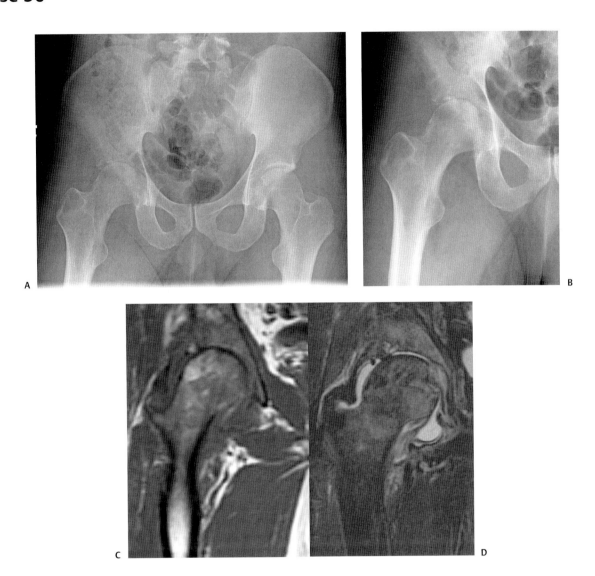

A

B

C

D

■ Clinical Presentation

A 40-year-old female presents with a 2-week history of severe atraumatic right hip pain.

■ Imaging Findings

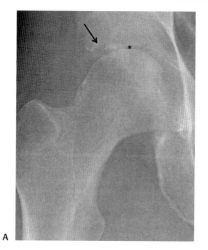
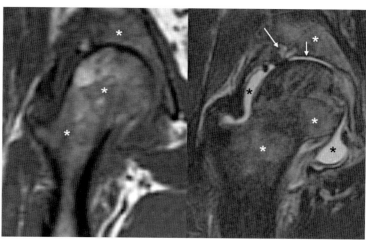

A   B, C

(A) Radiograph of the pelvis demonstrates asymmetric right hip superior and lateral joint space narrowing (*asterisk*) with periarticular osteopenia and acetabular erosions (*black arrow*). **(B)** Coronal fat-sensitive and **(C)** fluid-sensitive MR images through the right hip show a large effusion (*black asterisks*). Diffusely decreased T1 and increased T2 bone marrow signal intensity is seen throughout the femoral head/neck and acetabulum (*white asterisks*). Diffuse cartilage loss is seen about the acetabular roof and femoral head (*short white arrow*). Cystic erosive change involves the lateral margin of the acetabular roof (*long white arrow*).

■ Differential Diagnosis

- **Septic arthritis:** A monoarticular, atraumatic infectious process with corresponding imaging findings of erosions, effusion, joint space/cartilage loss, and periarticular osteopenia with profound bone marrow signal alteration on MRI.
- *Rheumatoid arthropathy:* A symmetric, erosive, polyarticular inflammatory arthropathy frequently causing severe acetabular protrusion of the bilateral hip joints.
- *Osteoarthritis:* A degenerative condition represented by superior and lateral femoral acetabular joint space narrowing and subchondral sclerosis with marginal osteophyte formation.

■ Essential Facts

- Septic arthritis and osteomyelitis in adults is usually related to hematogenous seeding from staphylococcal or streptococcal microorganisms.
- Infectious agents may also enter the joint by direct invasion from a penetrating wound, contiguous spread from adjacent soft tissues, or from a focus of osteomyelitis in the adjacent bone.
- Patients typically present with atraumatic, monoarticular pain and joint tenderness.
- Early radiographic changes of septic arthritis include periarticular osteopenia, joint effusion, and soft tissue swelling, with uniform joint space loss.

- Widening of the joint space may also be present in the setting of an effusion and/or synovial thickening.
- MRI findings of septic arthritis include a joint effusion with superimposed synovial thickening which demonstrates profound enhancement.
- MRI findings of diffuse cartilage thinning with underlying bony erosions may also be present.
- Bone marrow signal changes of osteomyelitis include decreased T1 and increased T2 signal intensity with associated enhancement.
- Treatment varies from antibiotic therapy to surgery, depending on the extent of the infection.

■ Other Imaging Findings

- The three-phase radionuclide bone scan is typically positive secondary to periarticular soft tissue inflammatory changes, synovial thickening, and osteomyelitis.

✓ Pearls and ✗ Pitfalls

- ✓ Hematogenous seeding by bloodborne pathogens is commonly seen in the S joints, which include the spine, sacroiliac joints, sternoclavicular joints, symphysis pubis, and shoulder (acromioclavicular joint).
- ✗ Radiographs may be negative in the acute stage of septic arthritis, necessitating joint aspiration.

Case 91

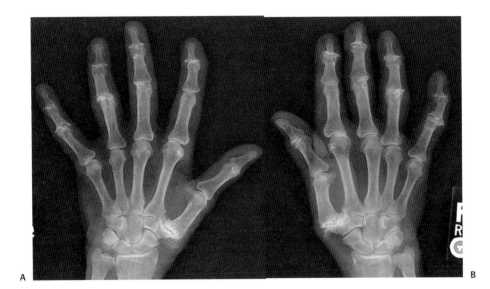

■ Clinical Presentation

An elderly female patient presents with pain and swelling over the proximal interphalangeal (PIP) and distal interphalangeal (DIPs) joints of both hands.

■ **Imaging Findings**

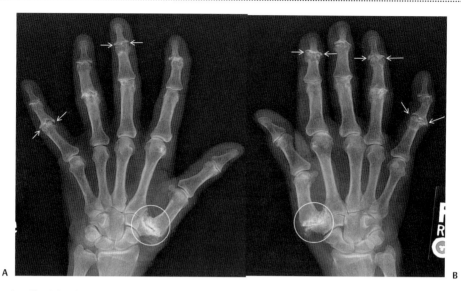

(A, B) Frontal radiographs of both hands show joint space narrowing with sclerosis and prominent marginal osteophyte formation at multiple interphalangeal (IP) joints. Subarticular erosive changes cause "gull-wing" deformities (*arrows*) at multiple IP joints. Also seen is marked joint space narrowing with exuberant osteophyte formation and subcortical cystic erosive change at both thumb carpometacarpal (CMC) joints (*encircled*).

■ **Differential Diagnosis**

- ***Erosive osteoarthritis:*** An inflammatory arthritic process causing bilateral interphalangeal (IP) joint osteoarthritic changes containing central subarticular erosions and subchondral bone plate collapse resembling seagull wings
- *Osteoarthrosis:* A degenerative process composed of joint space loss, sclerosis, and osteophyte formation localized to the distal IP joints of the hands.
- *Rheumatoid arthritis:* A symmetric, erosive inflammatory arthropathy that causes periarticular erosions, osteopenia, and subluxations at the metacarpophalangeal and PIP joints of the hands.

■ **Essential Facts**

- Erosive osteoarthritis represents a form of osteoarthritis that has a prominent element of synovitis and bony proliferation.
- The typical patient is a postmenopausal female with swelling, redness, and pain of the bilateral IP joints.
- Etiologies of this arthropathy include hormonal influences, a hereditary component, or an autoimmune process.

- The typical radiographic findings are similar to osteoarthrosis and include joint space loss secondary to cartilage loss. Subchondral sclerosis with exuberant osteophyte formation is typical for this arthropathy. Central subarticular erosions occur from underlying synovitis resulting in central articular depressions which cause a gull-wing appearance.
- Affected joints of the hand include the proximal and distal IP joints and, less commonly, the thumb CMC joint.
- The erosive changes may progress in a distal-to-proximal fashion at the level of the IP joints.

✓ **Pearls and ✗ Pitfalls**

✓ Osteopenia is a rare feature of this arthropathy, allowing distinction from rheumatoid arthritis.
✓ Persistent synovitis of the IP joints may progress to fusion.
✗ Gull-wing deformities may also be seen in patients with psoriatic arthritis.

Case 92

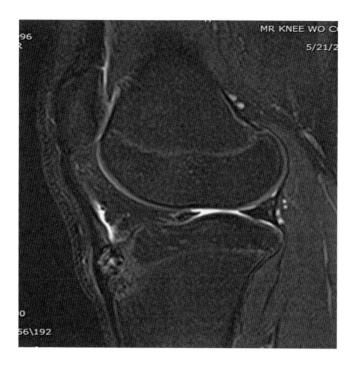

■ Clinical Presentation

An active adolescent male patient presents with pain and swelling inferior to the patella.

■ **Imaging Findings**

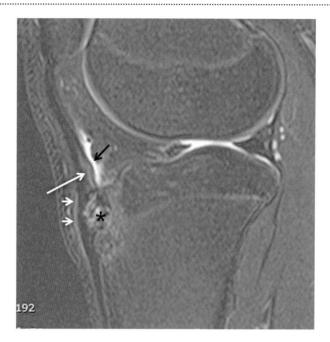

Sagittal fluid-sensitive MR image through the knee joint demonstrates bone marrow edema with osseous fragmentation at the level of the tibial tuberosity apophysis (*asterisk*). There is mild signal increase and thickening involving the distal patellar tendon (*long white arrow*). The deep infrapatellar bursa shows fluid distention (*black arrow*), and there is mild superficial infrapatellar edema (*short white arrows*).

■ **Differential Diagnosis**

• ***Osgood–Schlatter disease:*** A traction apophysitis affecting the tibial tuberosity.
• *Jumper's knee:* Proximal patellar tendinopathy secondary to overuse and repetitive traction.
• *Sinding–Larsen–Johansson disease:* An osseous avulsion injury of the inferior pole of the patella seen in the early adolescent patient.

■ **Essential Facts**

• Osgood–Schlatter disease represents a traction apophysitis at the patellar tendon–tibial tuberosity interface.
• This process is seen in active adolescents presenting with tenderness, swelling, and redness over the tibial tuberosity, and it may be bilateral in ~50% of patients.
• MR imaging reveals osseous cartilaginous edema at the level of the tibial tuberosity. T2 signal increase/ inflammation within the superficial and deep infrapatellar fat, along with thickening of the distal patellar tendon, is seen. Fluid distention of the deep infrapatellar bursa may be present.

• Osgood–Schlatter disease may have an association with patellofemoral malalignment and patella alta.
• Typical treatment includes anti-inflammatory medication along with physical therapy.

■ **Other Imaging Findings**

• Typical radiographic findings include soft tissue fullness over the tibial tuberosity with superimposed tibial tuberosity avulsive fragments and thickening of the patellar tendon.

✓ **Pearls and ✗ Pitfalls**

✓ Adult knee radiographs demonstrating an enlarged and/ or irregular tibial tuberosity with adjacent nonunited fragments likely represents sequela of this process.
✗ Acute tibial tuberosity avulsion fractures may occur in this patient subset, confounding the diagnosis.

Case 93

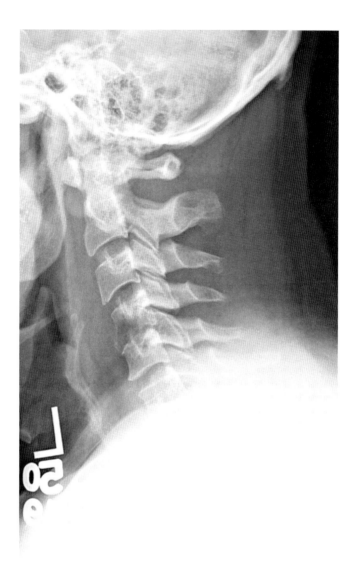

■ **Clinical Presentation**

A 40-year-old male patient presents with a 2-week history of insidious onset of atraumatic neck pain.

■ **Imaging Findings**

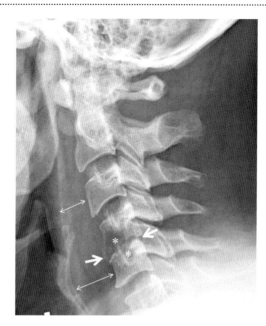

Lateral radiograph of the cervical spine demonstrates marked prevertebral soft tissue fullness (*double arrows*). C4–C5 intervertebral disk loss is seen (*arrows*), with end-plate erosive changes (*asterisks*).

■ **Differential Diagnosis**

- ***Spondylodiskitis:*** An infectious process involving the disk space and vertebral bodies causing localized vertebral body end-plate destruction with prevertebral soft tissue fullness.
- *Degenerative disk disease:* A degenerative process composed of intervertebral disk space narrowing, end-plate sclerosis, and osteophyte formation.
- *Amyloid spondyloarthropathy:* A chronic and asymptomatic form of spondylosis related to amyloid deposition typically seen in diabetics on long-term hemodialysis.

■ **Essential Facts**

- Spondylodiskitis represents an infectious process involving the disk and surrounding vertebral bodies.
- Hematogenous spread serves as the most common mode of inoculation.
- The most common pathogen is *Staphylococcus aureus.*
- Typical patient presentation is insidious onset of pain without relief from rest or analgesics.
- Associated risk factors include intravenous drug use, immunosuppression, diabetes, and advanced age.
- The vascularized intervertebral disk tissue serves as the initial origin of infection in the pediatric population, with eventual spread to the vertebral bodies.
- The anterior vertebral body serves as the initial site of inoculation in the adult spine, with subsequent spread to the disk space and adjoining vertebral body.

- Of the entire adult spine, the cervical spine is the least commonly affected.
- Classic radiographic findings of spondylodiskitis include intervertebral disk space loss, indistinction, and erosions of the vertebral body end-plates, with surrounding soft tissue swelling.
- Most spinal infections may be managed medically with antibiotic therapy.

■ **Other Imaging Findings**

- Radionuclide bone scans utilizing technetium-99m methylene diphosphonate and gallium are highly sensitive in the detection of spondylodiskitis and demonstrate increased isotope uptake.
- MRI findings of T2 hyperintensity with contrast enhancement at the disk space and within the adjacent vertebral bodies combined with adjacent abscess formation are characteristic.

✓ **Pearls and** ✗ **Pitfalls**

✓ Vacuum disk phenomenon is extremely rare in spondylodiskitis and virtually excludes this diagnosis.
✗ Normal radiographs do not exclude spondylodiskitis in the acute stage because radiographic changes may take up to 2 weeks to become visible.

Case 94

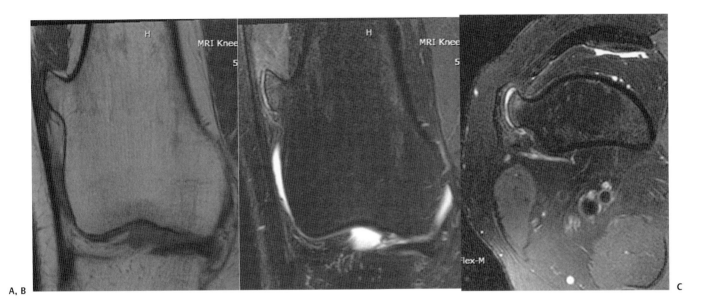

A, B

C

■ Clinical Presentation

A 35-year-old male patient presents with anterior and lateral knee joint pain.

■ **Imaging Findings**

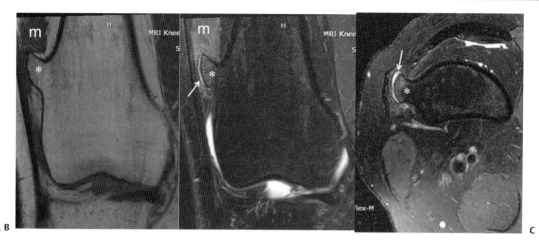

A, B　　C

(A–C) MR imaging of the knee joint utilizing coronal fat-sensitive **(A)**, coronal fluid-sensitive **(B)**, and axial fluid-sensitive **(C)** sequences demonstrates an osseous protuberance contiguous with the medullary canal extending from the lateral epicondyle of the distal femur (*asterisk*). This lesion indents the overlying quadriceps muscle belly (*m*), causing muscle edema. This protuberance contains minimal bone marrow edema. A T2-hyperintense, thin, < 1 cm, cartilaginous cap overlies this osseous protuberance (*arrow*).

■ **Differential Diagnosis**

- *Osteochondroma:* The most common benign cartilaginous neoplasm in the adult skeleton, represented by an osseous protuberance contiguous with the medullary canal containing a cartilaginous cap.

■ **Essential Facts**

- Osteochondroma, or exostosis, is the most common benign bone tumor in the adult skeleton.
- The origin of osteochondroma relates to a physeal cartilage migrational abnormality during enchondral ossification.
- The metaphyses of the long bones of the lower extremity are most frequently affected.
- Osteochondromas may be solitary or multiple, the latter being associated with the autosomal-dominant syndrome, multiple hereditary exostoses.
- The majority of solitary osteochondromas are asymptomatic and discovered incidentally.
- Symptoms typically relate to mass effect of the osteochondroma upon adjacent soft tissues.
- Characteristic features of osteochondroma include a sessile or pedunculated bony protuberance extending from the parent bone exhibiting cortical and medullary continuity with or without a calcified cartilaginous cap.
- MR imaging is the best modality for visualizing the effect of the lesion on surrounding structures and for evaluation of the cartilaginous cap.
- The thickness of the cartilaginous cap, as measured on MRI, is typically 1 to 3 cm in young patients and diminishes in size to < 1 cm in adult patients.

■ **Other Imaging Findings**

- Radiographs reveal a pedunculated or sessile bony excrescence extending from the parent long bone, with cortical medullary continuity. Chondroid calcifications within the cartilaginous cap may be detected.
- CT provides improved visualization of the cortex and medullary canal of the osteochondroma and its relationship with the parent bone. Chondroid calcifications are ideally evaluated with this imaging modality.

✓ **Pearls and** ✗ **Pitfalls**

- ✓ The typical growth pattern of osteochondroma is angulation away from the nearest joint secondary to mass effect from overlying tendons and ligaments.
- ✗ MR evaluation of the cartilage cap may be compromised by surrounding soft tissue inflammation and/or adventitial bursal formation.

Case 95

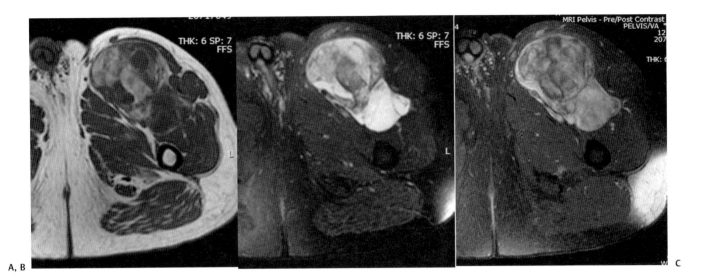

A, B
C

■ Clinical Presentation

A 50-year-old male patient presents with a painless thigh mass.

■ Imaging Findings

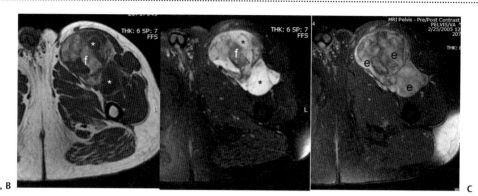

A, B

C

(A–C) Axial fat-sensitive **(A)**, fluid-sensitive **(B)**, and fat-suppressed postcontrast **(C)** MR images through the left thigh demonstrate a deep-seated, intramuscular, multiloculated mass within the quadriceps. Less than 50% of the lesion contains amorphous-appearing fat signal intensity (*f*). The majority of this mass contains cystlike fluid signal intensity (*asterisk*) with heterogeneous enhancement (*e*).

■ Differential Diagnosis

- ***Myxoid liposarcoma:*** A myxoid variant of liposarcoma containing a minor component of amorphous fat signal intensity upon a background of myxoid cystic-appearing components with intense heterogeneous enhancement.
- *Lipoma:* The most common benign soft tissue tumor in the adult skeleton demonstrating homogeneous fat signal intensity on MRI without nodularity, enhancement, or internal T2 signal increase.
- *Myxoma:* A well-defined, benign intramuscular mass exhibiting uniformly hypointense T1 and hyperintense T2 signal characteristics on MRI. This mass demonstrates mild heterogeneous enhancement and no internal fat signal intensity.

■ Essential Facts

- Myxoid liposarcoma represents the second most common subtype of liposarcoma.
- The mean age at presentation is 42 years of age, with complaint of a large, slow-growing, and painless mass.
- This lesion occurs most commonly in the lower extremity musculature and is rarely seen in the subcutaneous fat.
- Myxoid liposarcoma has an affinity for the thigh musculature.
- Histopathology reveals an abundance of myxoid matrix with arborizing vascularity and lipoblastic hypercellularity.
- Typical MR features include a multiloculated mass with a high myxomatous content demonstrating low T1 and high T2 signal intensity with profuse enhancement. Interposed foci of fat signal intensity are seen occupying ~10 to 25% of the entire tumor volume with a lacy, linear, or amorphous appearance.

■ Other Imaging Findings

- Ultrasound imaging demonstrates a complex, hypoechoic solid appearing mass helping to distinguish this lesion from a cystic mass.

✓ Pearls and ✗ Pitfalls

- ✓ Atypical metastases may occur in the paraspinal tissues, bone, retroperitoneum, and contralateral extremity.
- ✗ This neoplasm may exhibit no fat components on MR imaging, complicating the diagnosis.
- ✗ In the absence of gadolinium administration, these lesions may be misdiagnosed as large benign cysts.

Case 96

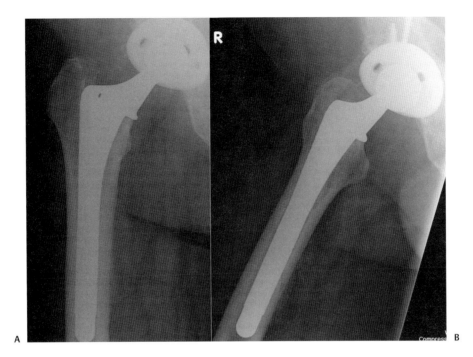

A

R

B

Compress

■ Clinical Presentation

A patient presents with right hip pain after stepping off of a curb.

■ Imaging Findings

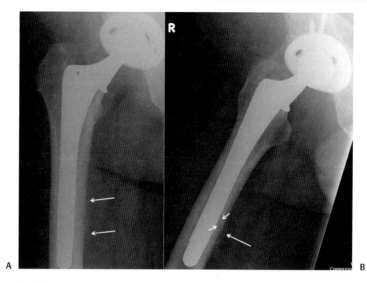

(A) Frontal and **(B)** lateral radiographs of the right hip demonstrate noncemented total hip arthroplasty changes. There is focal periosteal reaction (*long arrows*) along the medial femoral cortex at the level of the distal femoral prosthesis. A superimposed unicortical fracture is seen (*short arrows*).

■ Differential Diagnosis

- ***Periprosthetic fracture:*** Cortical interruption along the bone–hardware interface of an arthroplasty component is consistent with this diagnosis.

■ Essential Facts

- Hip arthroplasty postoperative periprosthetic fractures occur more commonly around the femur.
- These periprosthetic femoral fractures typically occur at the level of the femoral stem tip.
- This region serves as a stress riser caused by the difference in stiffness between the metal stem and native bone.
- This postoperative fracture typically occurs with minor trauma.
- Radiographic evaluation of hip arthroplasty components should include the entire femoral prosthesis.
- Radiographic findings include cortical interruption adjacent to the prosthetic component with or without superimposed periosteal reaction or fragment displacement/cortical offset.
- Intraoperative periprosthetic femoral fractures may occur in the peritrochanteric region.

■ Other Imaging Findings

- Dual-energy CT scanning is ideally suited to diagnose periprosthetic fractures. This technique allows photon energy optimization without prior knowledge of the prosthesis composition.

✓ Pearls and ✗ Pitfalls

- ✓ Pubic rami and sacral insufficiency fractures may develop in hip arthroplasty patients as a result of altered load transfer.
- ✗ A prominent vascular channel normally lies along the posterior medial cortex of the femur and may be mistaken for a periprosthetic fracture on radiographs or CT imaging.

Case 97

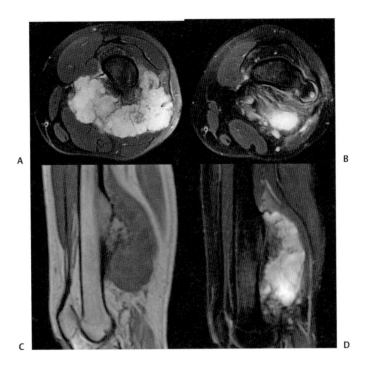

■ Clinical Presentation

A 25-year-old female patient with a history of "bone disorder" complains of posterior thigh pain and fullness of 2 months' duration.

■ Imaging Findings

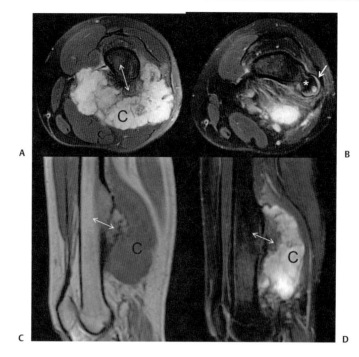

(A, B) MRI axial fluid-sensitive sequences along with sagittal **(C)** fat- and **(D)** fluid-sensitive sequences demonstrate a broad-based and irregular osseous excrescence extending from the posterior distal femoral diaphysis. This lesion exhibits at least partial continuity with the femoral medullary canal (*double arrows*). A thickened, irregular, lobulated, and peripherally expanding hyperintense T2 cartilage cap (C) overlies this osseous excrescence peripherally displacing the surrounding soft tissues. Imaging along the more distal femur demonstrates a smaller osseous excrescence also showing continuity with the cortex and medullary canal (*asterisk*) and containing a thin cartilaginous cap (*arrow*).

■ Differential Diagnosis

- **Chondrosarcoma (secondary to multiple hereditary exostosis):** A secondary chondroid sarcomatous lesion differentiating from an osteochondroma displaying a thickened, irregular cartilaginous cap.
- *Parosteal osteosarcoma:* A surface variant of osteosarcoma typically located along the posterior distal femur, characterized by irregular osteoid formation surrounded by a soft tissue mass without underlying medullary bone invasion.

■ Essential Facts

- Multiple hereditary exostosis, also known as *diaphyseal aclasis* or *multiple osteochondromatosis*, is an autosomal-dominant disorder characterized by two or more osteochondromas in the axial or appendicular skeleton.
- Transformation of these lesions to a chondrosarcoma may occur in ~2 to 5% of patients.
- The most common sites for malignant degeneration occur around the hip/shoulder joints and the bony pelvis.
- Clinical signs worrisome for malignant transformation include change in lesion size and/or insidious onset of pain after skeletal maturity.
- The malignant transformation occurs at the level of the cartilage component of the lesion with MRI demonstrating a hyperintense T2 cartilage cap with a lobular and aggressive peripheral growth pattern.
- A cartilaginous cap thickness of > 2 cm, suggests malignant transformation.
- Punctate chondroid calcifications manifesting as MRI signal voids may also be present.
- The vast majority of these chondrosarcomas are low grade and are treated by surgical excision.

✓ Pearls and ✕ Pitfalls

- ✓ Primary or secondary chondrosarcomas are extremely rare in the feet and hands.
- ✓ New onset of pain serves as the most helpful clinical determinant for malignant degeneration.
- ✕ Cystic adventitial bursal formation adjacent to osteochondromas may mimic a malignant soft tissue mass.

Case 98

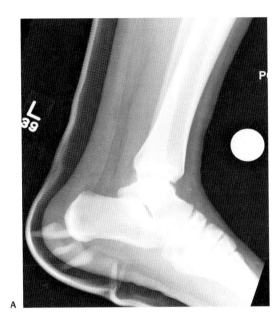

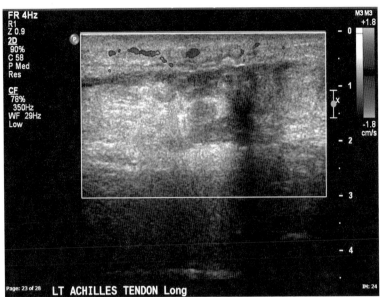

A

B

■ Clinical Presentation

A 31-year-old soccer player experiences severe pain behind the ankle while sprinting.

■ **Imaging Findings**

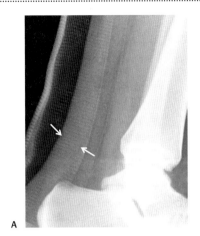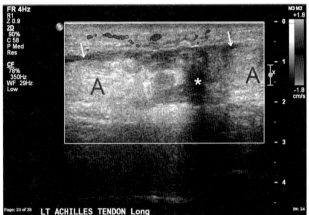

(A) Lateral radiograph of the ankle shows an overlying fiberglass splint in place. There is thickening of the Achilles tendon shadow (*arrows*) proximal to the calcaneal insertion. **(B)** Longitudinal ultrasound image of the Achilles tendon (*A*) shows loss of the normal fibrillar, linear echogenic tendon architecture with nonuniform and irregular tendon thickening. A hypoechoic defect (*asterisk*) extends through the Achilles tendon, with sonolucent fluid (*arrows*) surrounding the tendon. Acoustic shadowing is present deep to the Achilles tendon defect.

■ **Differential Diagnosis**

• **Achilles tendon rupture:** A traumatic tendon injury frequently seen in young adult males demonstrating thickening of the Achilles tendon shadow on radiographs. Ultrasound imaging demonstrating loss of the normal fibrillar tendon architecture with a hypoechoic tendon defect.

■ **Essential Facts**

• The Achilles tendon is derived from tendon fibers of the medial and lateral heads of the gastrocnemius and the soleus musculature and represents the strongest tendon of the human body, inserting on the posterior calcaneal tuberosity.
• Achilles tendon ruptures typically occur 2 to 6 cm proximal to the calcaneal insertion related to the relative hypovascularity of the tendon at this site. This region is referred to as the *critical zone* and is a common site for hypoxic degenerative tendon changes related to ischemia.
• These injuries are seen in younger patients with a mean age of 36 years and a male predominance. There is a significant relationship with leisure athletic activities such as running sports, particularly those that involve pivot and pushing-off maneuvers at the level of the foot and ankle.
• The normal Achilles tendon should be uniform in thickness and have a flat or concave anterior margin measuring no more than 5 mm in anterior posterior thickness.

• In the acute phase of a full-thickness tear, lateral radiographs of the ankle reveal loss of the normal pre-Achilles fat–tendon interface, with surrounding soft tissue swelling.
• Chronic interstitial tearing and tendinopathy of the Achilles tendon manifests with diffuse thickening of the Achilles tendon on lateral ankle radiographs.
• Disruption of the Achilles tendon is represented by hypoechoic or sonolucent changes through the Achilles tendon on ultrasound images.
• Peritendinitis may be seen as sonolucent fluid surrounding the perimeter of the Achilles tendon.
• Reporting of any associated tendon retraction is important for treatment purposes.

■ **Other Imaging Findings**

• MR findings include tendon discontinuity with interstitial tendon T2 signal increase and a fluid-filled tendon defect.

✓ **Pearls and ✗ Pitfalls**

✓ Posterior acoustic shadowing at the site of complete tendon rupture is commonly seen related to refraction of the ultrasound waves by the frayed and torn tendon edges.
✗ Artifactually decreased tendon echogenicity may occur if the ultrasound beam is not oriented perpendicular to the tendon fibers, referred to as *anisotropy*.

Case 99

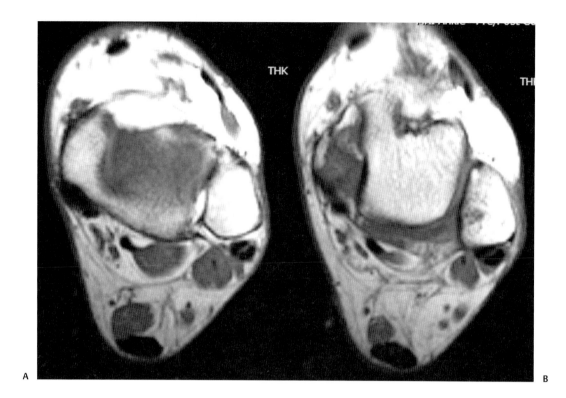

A

B

■ Clinical Presentation

An incidental finding on MRI of the ankle.

■ Imaging Findings

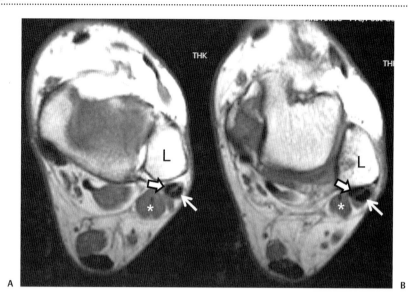

A   B

(A, B) Axial fat-sensitive MR images through the ankle at the level of the lateral malleolus (*L*) demonstrate a normal-appearing peroneus brevis (*thick block arrow*) and peroneus longus (*thin white arrow*). An accessory muscle belly lies posterior and medial to these tendons (*asterisk*).

■ Differential Diagnosis

- *Peroneus quartus:* An accessory muscle belly positioned posterior and medial to the peroneus brevis at the level of the lateral malleolus.

■ Essential Facts

- The peroneus quartus is the most frequently reported accessory peroneal muscle, with an estimated incidence of ~13 to 26%.
- This variant is typically bilateral and is common in males.
- The peroneus quartus originates at the level of the distal lateral fibula and descends medially and posteriorly.
- A frequent insertion site includes the calcaneal retrotrochlear eminence. Less common insertion sites include the fifth phalanx, the fifth metatarsal, the peroneal tendon, or the cuboid.

- Patients with this variant are typically asymptomatic. Crowding of the peroneal brevis tendon may occur, however, causing pain, swelling, tenosynovitis, tendon subluxation, or longitudinal interstitial tearing.
- MRI demonstrates an accessory tendon and muscle coursing posterior and medial to the peroneus brevis and peroneus longus.

✓ Pearls and ✗ Pitfalls

- ✓ This muscle is best demonstrated on axial images and is typically separated from the peroneus brevis muscle by a fat plane.
- ✗ The accessory peroneus quartus may be mistaken for a peroneus brevis tendon split tear.

Case 100

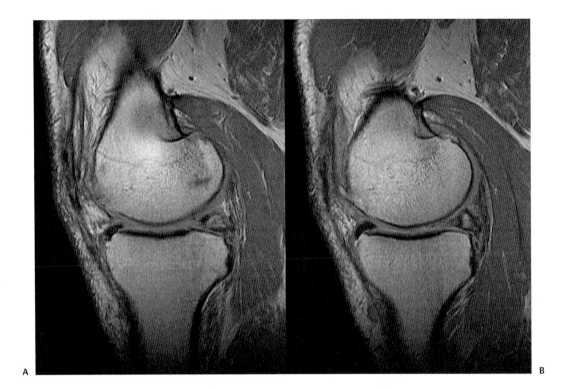

■ Clinical Presentation

A patient presents with a remote history of trauma and suspected internal derangement.

■ Imaging Findings

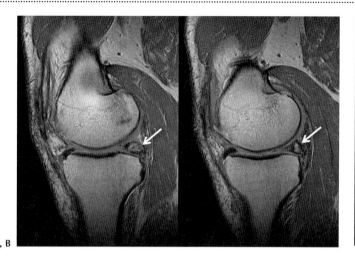 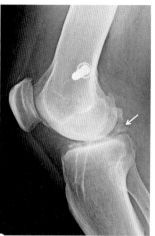

A, B   **C**

(A, B) Sagittal fat-sensitive MR images through the medial meniscus demonstrate a hyperintense rounded/triangular structure embedded within the posterior horn medial meniscus (*arrows*). **(C)** A lateral knee radiograph of the same patient demonstrates a triangular ossific density superimposed over the expected location of the posterior horn medial meniscus (*arrow*). Anterior cruciate ligament (ACL) reconstructive changes are also demonstrated.

■ Differential Diagnosis

- ***Meniscal ossicle:*** Bone formation within meniscal tissue.
- *Loose body (secondary synovial osteochondromatosis):* A process associated with osteoarthritis which involves ossification of fragments of hyaline cartilage shed from the articular surface of a joint.
- *Sesamoid bone:* A congenital focus of ossification seen within tendons.

■ Essential Facts

- Meniscal ossicle represents bone formation typically seen within the posterior horn medial meniscus which may progress with time.
- This finding may be associated with posterior horn medial meniscal root disruption and trauma.
- This ossicle is uncommon with < 1% incidence.

■ Other Imaging Findings

- Detectable on CT scan as an ossific density in meniscal tissue.

✓ Pearls and ✗ Pitfalls

- ✓ May assume a triangular appearance on radiographs related to the posterior horn meniscal morphology.
- ✓ MRI fat-sensitive sequences are essential for identification of fat within the ossicle.
- ✗ Loose osseous/chondral bodies frequently lie adjacent to the posterior meniscal horns and may mimic a meniscal ossicle.

Case Questions and Answers

The questions and answers in the following section are numbered as cases 1 through 100. The questions correspond to the respectively numbered case reviews and are intended to be answered after working through the cases.

■ **Case 1**

1. All of the following statements regarding bisphosphonate fractures are true except...
   a) Most patients on bisphosphonate therapy for osteoporosis will not experience this complication.
   b) Bisphosphonates suppress osteoclast activity and inhibit bone resorption.
   c) The typical duration of drug use before this complication arises is ~1 year.
   d) Patients with bisphosphonate fractures may require femoral orthopedic hardware stabilization.

The correct answer is (**c**). The average duration of bisphosphonate usage before potentially developing insufficiency fractures is ~7 years.

2. What is the proposed mechanism by which these fractures occur?
   a) Oversuppression of bone turnover and suppressed bony remodeling resulting in skeletal fragility
   b) Blockage of intestinal vitamin D resorption
   c) Phosphate wasting
   d) Failure of vitamin D hydroxylation

The correct answer is (**a**). Extended bisphosphonate therapy is believed to inhibit bone turnover and remodeling, resulting in increased skeletal fragility.

■ **Case 2**

1. Regarding the acoustic shadowing of a foreign body, which of the following statements is true?
   a) Foreign body composition determines the extent of shadowing.
   b) Surface contour is the primary determinant of acoustic shadowing.
   c) Foreign body acoustic shadowing is always present.
   d) None of the above is true.

The correct answer is (**b**). Shadowing artifacts from foreign bodies is dependent upon the surface contour of the foreign body rather than the foreign body composition. Smooth and flat surfaces produce dirty shadowing, whereas irregular surfaces with a small radius produce clean shadowing. Not all foreign bodies cause acoustic shadowing.

2. Primary advantages of ultrasound evaluation of foreign bodies compared with other imaging modalities include which of the following?
   a) Affordability
   b) Lack of radiation
   c) Availability
   d) Portability
   e) All of the above

The correct answer is (**e**). Ultrasound imaging has become the standard of care for evaluation of superficial foreign body detection. Features that make ultrasound imaging the ideal choice include its affordability, portability, availability, and absence of irradiation.

■ **Case 3**

1. Demonstration of a meniscal flounce requires which of the following?
   a) Imaging of the contralateral knee given the increased incidence of bilaterality
   b) Increased suspicion for meniscocapsular injury and other ligamentous injuries
   c) Detailed description with implication of a superimposed meniscal tear
   d) MR arthrography

The correct answer is (**b**). The majority of cases of meniscal flounce relate to a normal variant secondary to positioning. However, a diligent search for coexisting pathology is mandatory when flouncing is detected, given that ligamentous injury, meniscal tears, and capsular laxity may exaggerate this wrinkling phenomenon.

2. Theoretically, injury to all of the following structures may lead to lateral meniscal flouncing except...
   a) Anterior inferior popliteal meniscal fascicle
   b) Posterior superior popliteal meniscal fascicle
   c) Ligament of Wrisberg
   d) Lateral collateral ligament (LCL)
   e) Meniscal homologue

The correct answer is (**e**). The popliteal meniscal fascicles, the LCL, and the meniscal femoral ligaments have an intimate association with the lateral meniscus and are important for its functioning and stability. As a result, injury to these structures may result in altered mobility of the lateral meniscus predisposing to flouncing. The meniscal homologue is located in the wrist and serves as a stabilizer of the ulnar collateral ligament complex.

■ Case 4

1. Regarding wrist arthrography, which of the following is true?
   a) A 25-gauge needle is the best choice for injection.
   b) The ideal injection volume for the distal radial ulnar joint (DRUJ) is 1 to 2 mL.
   c) The ideal injection volume for the radiocarpal joint is 8 to 10 mL.
   d) None of the above
   e) Both a and b

The correct answer is (**e**). The ideal volume of injection for the radiocarpal compartment is 3 to 4 mL. The ideal injection volume for the distal radial ulnar joint (DRUJ) is 1 to 2 mL. The optimal needle size is a 25-gauge needle which minimizes patient discomfort. Additionally, wrist arthrography injections should avoid the site of symptoms in an effort to prevent iatrogenic disruption of the normal anatomy from the injection.

2. The optimal MR arthrography sequences for wrist internal derangements include all of the following except…
   a) T1 fat-suppressed images
   b) T2 fat-suppressed images
   c) Thin-slice 3D dual-echo steady-state precession (DESSP)
   d) Diffusion-weighted imaging

The correct answer is (**d**). Diffusion-weighted imaging has no role in TFC imaging. Fat-suppressed T1-weighted imaging is designed to provide optimal contrast resolution on MR arthrography. T2-weighted fat-suppressed imaging allows detection of bone marrow abnormalities. Thin-slice 3D DESSP imaging allows detailed analysis of the thin ligaments of the wrist.

3. Regarding triangular fibrocartilage (TFC) tears, which of the following statements is true?
   a) Tears frequently occur through the membranous segment.
   b) Pseudo-tears may occur adjacent to the radial attachment.
   c) Tears along the ulnar attachment have a favorable outcome given increased vascularity.
   d) All of the above are true.

The correct answer is (**d**). TFC tears frequently occur through the membranous segment and tend to be symptomatic if they occur along the undersurface. TFC pseudo-tears may be erroneously diagnosed secondary to volume averaging between the hyaline cartilage of the distal radius and the radial insertional fibers of the TFC. Given the hypervascularity of the ulnar insertional fibers of the TFC, this segment of the TFC exhibits optimal healing.

■ Case 5

1. Which of the following statements is true regarding desmoid tumors?
   a) Notorious for local recurrence after resection
   b) Thought to be associated with pregnancy and trauma
   c) Typically painless lesion
   d) No metastatic potential
   e) All of the above are true

The correct answer is (**e**). Desmoid tumors are frequently seen in women of childbearing age and may have an association with trauma. This relatively painless neoplasm can have a high level of local recurrence after resection. There have been no reported cases of metastasis associated with desmoid tumors.

2. All of the following are potential treatment options for desmoid tumors except…
   a) Wide local excision
   b) Radiation therapy
   c) Laser ablation
   d) Chemotherapy

The correct answer is (**c**). The most widely accepted treatment option for desmoid tumors is wide local excision, which minimizes chances of recurrence. Radiation therapy has been utilized for recurrent lesions and lesions located in anatomically complex locations. Success has been seen with variable chemotherapeutic regimens, particularly in patients with Gardner's syndrome. Laser ablation therapy is not a recognized form of desmoid treatment to date.

■ Case 6

1. All of the following may be seen on radiographs of patients with renal osteodystrophy except…
   a) Sacroiliac joint erosions
   b) Rugger jersey spine
   c) Diffuse skeletal sclerosis
   d) High-riding humeral heads
   e) "Salt-and-pepper" appearance of the skull

The correct answer is (**d**). High-riding humeral heads is a finding that coexists with rotator cuff tearing. This is frequently seen in patients with rheumatoid arthritis and calcium pyrophosphate dihydrate (CPPD) arthropathy. Sacroiliac joint subchondral erosions are a common feature of renal osteodystrophy. Additionally, bandlike sclerosis along the vertebral body end plates is another feature seen with this diagnosis and is referred to as rugger jersey spine. Calvarial trabecular bone resorption results in a "salt-and-pepper" appearance to the skull. Sclerotic changes within the skeleton may also be seen with renal osteodystrophy.

2. Expected imaging findings of patients with renal osteodystrophy include all of the following except...
   a) Renal atrophy
   b) Extensive vascular calcifications
   c) Extensive temporal lobe sclerosis
   d) Pericapsular juxta-articular calcific deposits

The correct answer is (**c**). Sclerosis of the temporal lobes of the brain is not a feature of this disease. However, the calcium and phosphate derangements associated with renal osteodystrophy account for the vascular and soft tissue metastatic calcific deposits. Additionally, the primary insult driving the pathophysiology of renal osteodystrophy is chronic renal disease, with renal atrophy frequently demonstrated on imaging.

■ Case 7

1. The characteristic soft tissue findings associated with this disease process may be best described by which of the following?
   a) Particle disease
   b) Aseptic lymphocytic vasculitis–associated lesion (ALVAL)
   c) Caseating necrosis
   d) Chronic granulomatous disease

The correct answer is (**b**). Although a component of metallosis and synovial thickening may coexist with this disease process, the primary feature of the soft tissue changes from these metallic particles is best described microscopically as ALVAL.

2. All of the following MR sequence adjustments may optimize evaluation of soft tissues adjacent to total hip arthroplasty (THA) hardware except...
   a) Decrease echo train length
   b) Decreased voxel size
   c) Increase receiver bandwidth
   d) 3T field strength
   e) Inversion recovery fat suppression (STIR)
   f) Thin sections

The correct answer is (**d**). Metal artifact reduction sequences (MARS) involve minimizing the effects of susceptibility artifact from the metallic hardware in place. These effects include signal voids, spatial misregistration, and uneven fat saturation. These artifacts are directly related to magnetic field strength. Therefore, 3-Tesla MR imaging is not recommended.

■ Case 8

1. Patients with ischiofemoral impingement may also suffer from which of the following?
   a) Sciatica
   b) Piriformis syndrome
   c) Meralgia paresthetica
   d) Ischial bursitis

The correct answer is (**a**). The quadratus femoris muscle extends from the posterior proximal medial femur to the lateral ischium and lies in close proximity to the sciatic nerve. As a result of this relationship, patients may exhibit sciatic nerve symptoms. The other listed diagnoses are not associated with ischiofemoral impingement.

2. Potential causes of ischiofemoral impingement include all of the following except...
   a) Trauma
   b) Lesser trochanter enthesophyte formation
   c) Congenital
   d) Osteoarthrosis
   e) Cam morphology of the femur

The correct answer is (**e**). Multiple proposed etiologies for this type of impingement include the widened female pelvis, lesser trochanter enthesophyte formation, osteoarthrosis, and posttraumatic remodeling of the ischium or proximal femur. However, cam-type femoral morphology is associated with femoral acetabular impingement and has no association with ischiofemoral impingement.

■ Case 9

1. All of the following are true regarding the cyclops lesion except...
   a) This lesion derives its name from its bulbous appearance resembling an eye.
   b) The typical cyclops lesion ranges in size from 10 to 15 mm.
   c) Most cyclops lesions are visible on radiographs.
   d) A name frequently interchanged with the cyclops lesion is arthrofibrosis.

The correct answer is (**c**). The cyclops lesion is readily diagnosed on MRI and is not visible on radiography. The cyclops lesion derives its name from the arthroscopic resemblance of the lesion to the mythical one-eyed cyclops monster. Anterior arthrofibrosis is another descriptive term for this lesion. The typical lesion size ranges from 1.0 to 1.5 cm.

2. Which of the following is true regarding the cyclops lesion?
    a) The risk of developing a cyclops lesion may be increased if the anterior edge of the tibial tunnel lies anterior to a line drawn along the intercondylar roof in the sagittal plane with the knee fully extended.
    b) An increased risk of a cyclops lesion has been reported in remnant-preserving anterior cruciate ligament (ACL) repair techniques.
    c) Tissues found within the cyclops lesion may include fibrocartilaginous tissue, synovium, and fat.
    d) All of the above statements are true.

The correct answer is (**d**). All of the listed statements are true. Graft impingement from the anterior tibial tunnel malpositioning has been implicated with the cyclops lesion. Remnant-preserving ACL repair techniques present an increased risk of cyclops lesions. Fibrocartilaginous tissue, along with synovium and fat, have been described within this lesion.

■ Case 10

1. All of the following structures play an important role in securing the biceps tendon within the biceps sulcus except…
    a) The transverse humeral ligament
    b) The coracohumeral ligament
    c) The superior fibers of the subscapularis tendon
    d) The anterior fibers of the supraspinatus tendon
    e) The posterior band of the inferior glenohumeral ligament

The correct answer is (**e**). The above-listed structures are contained within the rotator interval and help stabilize the biceps tendon with the exception of the posterior band of the inferior glenohumeral ligament. The superior glenohumeral ligament is also included within the rotator interval and plays an important role for securing the proximal biceps tendon.

2. All of the following statements are true regarding the biceps tendon except…
    a) The biceps tendon sheath communicates with the glenohumeral joint.
    b) The biceps tendon is intra-articular but extrasynovial.
    c) The subscapularis tendon is an important medial stabilizer for the long head of the biceps tendon.
    d) Subscapularis tendon tears are most commonly associated with instability of the long head of the biceps tendon.
    e) All of the above statements are true.

The correct answer is (**e**). All of the listed statements are true. The biceps tendon sheath communicates with

the glenohumeral joint and may become distended with fluid in the setting of the glenohumeral joint effusion. The biceps tendon is an extrasynovial and intra-articular structure. The subscapularis muscle and tendon, along with the pectoralis muscle and tendon, help provide stability for the biceps tendon. Subscapularis tendon tears are commonly associated with instability of the long head of the biceps tendon.

■ Case 11

1. Regarding the Romanus lesion, which of the following statements is true?
    a) Represents a trauma-induced lesion of the vertebral body
    b) An inflammatory-based lesion centered along the ligamentum flavum
    c) An inflammatory-based lesion centered at the anterior and/or posterior edges of the vertebral body end plates
    d) An infectious lesion frequently superimposed upon spinal changes from ankylosing spondylitis (AS).

The correct answer is (**c**). The Romanus lesion represents a form of spondylitis described in the seronegative spondyloarthropathies. This lesion is best detected on lateral spinal radiographs consisting of erosive irregularity along the anterior and posterior edges of the vertebral body end plates. These changes may progress to sclerosis and have been termed "shiny corners," manifesting with bright T2 signal on MR imaging. These changes are secondary to spondylitis occurring at the attachment site of the annulus fibrosis to the vertebral end plate.

2. Regarding the Andersson lesion, which of the following statements is true?
    a) This lesion serves as a precursor to infectious diskitis.
    b) This represents a sterile inflammatory process related to the intervertebral disks.
    c) This lesion is typically seen in seronegative and seropositive inflammatory conditions.
    d) This represents a mechanical and degenerative process.

The correct answer is (**b**). The Andersson lesion represents a form of noninfectious diskitis seen with seronegative spondyloarthropathies. This process involves inflammation of the intervertebral disks seen in ~8% of patients with AS. This process may involve erosive changes extending into the superior end plate, inferior end plate, or both end plates of the vertebral body. Radiographs exhibit irregularity and erosion along the central portion of the vertebral body end plates with corresponding MRI signal changes of hyperintense T2 signal with a hemispheric appearance.

■ Case 12

1. All of the following locations may exhibit gouty erosions except…
    a) Patella
    b) Tarsal bones
    c) Carpometacarpal joints
    d) Spine
    e) All of the above

The correct answer is (**e**). Although gout was originally described as an appendicular skeletal crystalline arthropathy more frequently seen in the lower extremities, axial skeleton involvement may be seen in as many as 35% of cases. Sites of involvement in the axial skeleton may include the facet joints, the intervertebral disk spaces, and the atlantoaxial interval.

2. Radiographic findings seen with gout include the following:
    a) Relative preservation of joint spaces
    b) Intraosseous calcific deposits
    c) Intraosseous cystic lesions
    d) Tarsometatarsal joint erosions
    e) All of the above

The correct answer is (**e**). All of the listed radiographic findings are found. A hallmark finding for gouty arthritis is preservation of joint spaces. Gout may cause intraosseous lytic lesions with or without uric acid crystalline deposits. Intraosseous lytic gouty lesions are well described in the hands and patella. It is not uncommon for gouty erosions to affect the tarsometatarsal joints in the presence or absence of first metatarsal phalangeal joint erosions.

■ Case 13

1. Regarding the superior peroneal retinaculum, which of the following statements is false?
    a) Functions as a secondary restraint preventing peroneal tendon subluxation
    b) Anteriorly attaches to and blends with the fibular periosteum
    c) Rupture of this structure may or may not coexist with a lateral malleolus avulsion
    d) Serves as a secondary restraint to anterior and lateral ankle instability
    e) Posteriorly attaches to the Achilles tendon and calcaneus

The correct answer is (**a**). The superior peroneal retinaculum functions as the primary restrainer of peroneal tendon subluxation with the inferior peroneal retinaculum serving as the secondary restrainer. The superior peroneal retinaculum attaches anteriorly to the fibular periosteum and posteriorly to the Achilles tendon

and calcaneus. The majority of patients with superior peroneal retinacular avulsion and peroneal tendon subluxation will not have a lateral malleolus avulsion. This retinaculum serves as a secondary restrainer to anterior and lateral ankle stability.

2. All of the following may serve as potential causes for lateral peroneal subluxation except…
    a) Maisonneuve fracture
    b) Calcaneal fractures
    c) Hindfoot valgus deformities
    d) Answers a, b, and c
    e) Answers b and c

The correct answer is (**a**). Maisonneuve or pronation external rotation fractures typically do not implicate the superior peroneal retinaculum. Calcaneal fractures which exhibit excessive lateral wall bulging predispose to lateral peroneal tendon subluxation given the close proximity of the tendons to this segment of the calcaneus. Hindfoot valgus deformities also contribute to peroneal tendon subluxation related to the excessive lateral traction from this malalignment.

■ Case 14

1. Which of the following statements is true regarding the iliopsoas bursa?
    a) Fluid distention of this bursa should not normally be seen.
    b) The iliopsoas bursa is bilateral in the majority of patients.
    c) This bursa may serve as a route for the spread of infection.
    d) All of the above are true.
    e) None of the above is true.

The correct answer is (**d**). Fluid distention of the iliopsoas bursa is not normally seen and should be considered pathologic. The iliopsoas bursa is bilateral in the majority (~95%) of patients. The iliopsoas bursa may serve as a route for the spread of infection, particularly in the setting of a psoas muscle abscess, which may enable distal extension to the hip joint.

2. Which of the following statements is true?
    a) The iliopsoas bursa communicates with the hip joint in ~15% of patients secondary to degenerative capsular weakening.
    b) A proposed pathogenesis for iliopsoas bursitis is fluid/synovial herniation from a distended hip joint afflicted with osteoarthritis.
    c) Neither a nor b is true.
    d) Both a and b are true.

The correct answer is (**d**). Iliopsoas bursal communication with the hip joint can be seen in ~15% of patients. This likely results from degenerative weakening of the capsule related to underlying hip arthropathy. One proposed mechanism for iliopsoas bursitis is fluid and synovial herniation from a pressurized and arthritic hip joint.

■ Case 15

1. Which of the following statements is false regarding distal intersection syndrome?
   a) Intersection syndrome is more common than distal intersection syndrome.
   b) Distal intersection syndrome has been reported in skiers.
   c) Lister's tubercle is a dorsal cortical bony prominence extending from the distal radius separating the first and second extensor tendon compartments.
   d) A potential watershed zone exists about the extensor pollicis longus tendon adjacent to the distal intersection possibly contributing to the diagnosis.

The correct answer is (**c**). Lister's tubercle is a dorsal cortical bony prominence extending from the distal radius positioned between the second and third extensor compartment tendons. Intersection syndrome is reported to be more common than distal intersection syndrome. Distal intersection syndrome has been reported in skiers. One causative factor for distal intersection syndrome may relate to the paucity of blood supply of the extensor pollicis longus tendon predisposing to tendinopathy and tenosynovitis at the distal intersection.

2. All of the following statements are true regarding distal intersection syndrome except…
   a) The second and third extensor tendon compartments intersect distal to the radiocarpal joint.
   b) The extensor retinaculum may contribute to this diagnosis.
   c) The second and third extensor compartment tendons communicate with each other in the area of intersection.
   d) The extensor pollicis longus tendon travels deep to the second extensor compartment tendons.

The correct answer is (**d**). The second and third extensor tendons intersect distal to the radial carpal joint. The extensor retinaculum may serve as an aggravating factor for the development of tenosynovitis of these tendon sheaths. A communication exists between the second and third extensor compartment tendon sheaths. The extensor pollicis longus tendon travels superficial to the second extensor compartment tendons.

■ Case 16

1. Regarding the carpal boss:
   a) Patients may become symptomatic from this finding related to extensor tendon slippage over this bony prominence.
   b) The major axis of stress through the wrist occurs through the second and third carpometacarpal (CMC) junctions contributing to this finding.
   c) This may be seen in boxers related to repetitive axial loading along the longitudinal axis of the metacarpals.
   d) All of the above are true.
   e) None of the above is true.

The correct answer is (**d**). Patients with a carpal boss may become symptomatic related to extensor tendon slippage over this bony excrescence. A contributory factor to the development of the carpal boss relates to the primary stress transmission through the second and third CMC junctions. The boxing wrist is particularly prone to development of this ossicle.

2. Which of the following statements is false?
   a) The carpal boss may be entirely isolated, partially contiguous, or entirely continuous with the surrounding bony structures.
   b) The carpal boss is most commonly fused to the capitate.
   c) The carpal boss is more frequently seen in the right wrist.
   d) The carpal boss is most commonly fused to the second and third metacarpal bases.

The correct answer is (**b**). The carpal boss may be completely isolated or partially or entirely incorporated with the surrounding osseous structures. The carpal boss is most commonly fused to the second and third metacarpal bases. A carpal boss is more frequently seen in the right wrist, given the population predominance of right handedness.

■ Case 17

1. Potential indications for hip arthrography include:
   a) Assess for labral tears
   b) Optimize hyaline cartilage evaluation
   c) Evaluate for capsular laxity
   d) Diagnosis of avascular necrosis
   e) All of the above
   f) Answers a, b, and c

The correct answer is (**f**). MR arthrography is ideally suited to diagnose labral tears, hyaline cartilage defects, and capsular laxity. Hip arthrography is not required for the diagnosis of avascular necrosis.

2. An alternative to ensure intracapsular needle tip placement includes which of the following?
   a) Synovial fluid aspiration
   b) Hemorrhagic fluid aspiration
   c) Needle tip contact with the intracapsular cortical bone
   d) Decreased resistance when injecting anesthetic

The correct answer is (**a**). Synovial fluid is produced by the synovial membrane which lines the joint capsule. As a result, synovial fluid aspiration typically ensures intracapsular needle tip placement. Hemorrhagic fluid aspiration may relate to blood vessel injury and not necessarily intra-articular needle placement. Needle tip contact with the intracapsular cortical bone does not ensure the injected medicine will accumulate within the joint capsule. Variations of capsular insertion onto the femoral neck may be seen or the hip capsule may be collapsed, tight, or inflamed, limiting intracapsular access. Decreased resistance to injection of anesthetic does not ensure intracapsular needle tip placement, as this may occur with bursal or intramuscular fluid injection.

■ **Case 18**

1. Manifestations of hydroxyapatite deposition disease (HADD) include all of the following except...
   a) Silent phase
   b) Adhesive periarthritis phase
   c) Destructive intra-articular phase
   d) Infectious phase
   e) Mechanical phase

The correct answer is (**d**). Various phases and manifestations of HADD have been defined. A silent phase has been described in which patients are relatively asymptomatic and the crystalline deposits are well-organized on imaging. A mechanical phase occurs in which patients present with limited range of motion. Imaging during this phase shows partial resorption and redistribution of calcific deposits into adjacent bursae and bone. The adhesive periarthritis stage causes severe limited range of motion and pain with bursitis. An intra-articular manifestation of hydroxyapatite deposition manifests in the older patient as a rapidly destructive arthritis. An infectious phase of HADD does not exist.

2. Hydroxyapatite crystals have been identified in all of the following locations except...
   a) Bursa
   b) Meninges
   c) Cortical bone
   d) Collateral ligaments
   e) Medullary bone

The correct answer is (**b**). Hydroxyapatite crystalline deposition has been described in a variety of locations. The most common location of this deposit is within tendons. Other sites of deposition include cortical bone, the medullary canal, bursae, musculature, and collateral ligaments. Hydroxyapatite crystalline deposition has not been described within the meninges.

■ **Case 19**

1. The common extensor tendon and lateral epicondyle have contributions from all of the following muscles except...
   a) Extensor carpi radialis brevis
   b) Extensor carpi ulnaris
   c) Pronator teres
   d) Extensor digiti minimi
   e) Extensor digitorum communis

The correct answer is (**c**). The extensor carpi radialis brevis, extensor digitorum communis, and extensor carpi ulnaris form a conjoined tendon that attaches along the anterior aspect of the lateral epicondyle. This attachment is adjacent to the origins of the extensor carpi radialis longus and brachioradialis. The lateral epicondyle also serves as the site of attachment for the extensor digiti minimi. The pronator teres does not contribute to the common extensor tendon muscle mass and attaches to the medial epicondyle.

2. Associated injuries with severe common extensor tendinopathy and tearing may include which of the following?
   a) Radial collateral ligament injury
   b) Annular ligament injury
   c) Capsular injury
   d) Lateral ulnar collateral ligament injury
   e) All of the above

The correct answer is (**e**). Capsular injury as well as thickening and tearing of the lateral ulnar collateral ligament, radial collateral ligament, and annular ligament have been associated with severe common extensor tendinopathy and tearing. This association is related to the proximity of these ligamentous structures which are positioned just deep to the common extensor tendon.

■ **Case 20**

1. Which of the following findings may be seen in conjunction with posterior labral tears?
   a) Posterior capsular stripping, anterior humeral head impaction fractures, posterior humeral head subluxation
   b) Capsular laxity
   c) Inferior glenohumeral ligament injury
   d) Adhesive capsulitis
   e) Answers a, b, and c

The correct answer is (**e**). Posterior capsular stripping and laxity, humeral avulsion of the inferior glenohumeral ligament, along with posterior humeral head subluxation may be seen with posterior labral tearing resulting from trauma to the shoulder joint. A "trough sign" or reverse Hill–Sachs lesion is an impaction fracture positioned over the anterior aspect of the humeral head related to posterior shoulder dislocations. Adhesive capsulitis relates to an idiopathic inflammatory capsulitis, not typically associated with posterior labral tearing.

2. All of the following statements are true regarding the glenoid labrum except…
   a) Increases the depth and surface area of the glenoid fossa
   b) Significantly contributes to the stability of the glenohumeral joint
   c) Is primarily composed of hyaline cartilage
   d) Is ideally evaluated with MR arthrography
   e) Has a relationship with the long head of the biceps tendon

The correct answer is (**c**). The glenohumeral joint, a ball-and-socket joint, is inherently unstable secondary to the limited contact surface area between the humeral head and bony glenoid. The glenoid labrum significantly improves the stability of this articulation by increasing the depth and surface area of this articulation. The glenoid labrum is composed of fibrocartilage and is ideally evaluated with MR arthrography. The long head of the biceps tendon originates at the superior mid-point of the labrum at the level of the supraglenoid tubercle.

■ Case 21

1. Characteristics of elastofibroma include all of the following except…
   a) No malignant potential
   b) Estimated to be normally present in up to 2% of the population
   c) Equally distributed in men and women
   d) Typically found deep to the serratus anterior and latissimus dorsi musculature
   e) All of the above statements are true.

The correct answer is (**c**). Elastofibroma has no malignant potential. Rarely, recurrence is seen following resection secondary to incomplete resection. The reported occurrence in the general population is estimated at 2%, with females affected 5 to 13 times more than males. These lesions are typically seen adjacent to the serratus anterior and latissimus dorsi musculature in an infrascapular location.

2. Regarding imaging characteristics of elastofibroma, which of the following is false?
   a) Superimposed streaks of fat may be found within these lesions.
   b) A well-defined capsule is typical of these lesions.
   c) Ultrasound imaging displays multilayered hypoechoic layers of fat and fibrous tissue.
   d) These lesions have a variable enhancement pattern.

The correct answer is (**b**). Frequently, fatty streaks are noted within these lesions and are ideally displayed on MR and CT imaging. These lesions exhibit ill-defined margins interlaced with fat without a distinct capsule. Ultrasound imaging displays multiple echogenic layers consistent with the fat and fibrous tissue components. No consistent enhancement pattern has been observed with these lesions.

■ Case 22

1. Which of the following statements is true regarding meniscal root tears?
   a) Insufficiency fractures related to posterior horn medial meniscus root tears are more commonly seen in the medial tibial plateau.
   b) Anterior horn medial meniscus root tears are similar in frequency to posterior horn root tears.
   c) Peripheral meniscal body extrusion is only associated with meniscal root tears.
   d) None of the above statements is true.

The correct answer is (**d**). When present with medial meniscus root tears, insufficiency fractures are more commonly seen within the medial femoral condyle. The anterior horn of the medial meniscus is the least common area of meniscal tearing. Peripheral meniscal body extrusion may be seen with intrameniscal degenerative changes in the absence of meniscal root disruption.

2. Regarding meniscal anatomy, which of the following statements is true?
   a) Four major meniscal root anchors exist.
   b) The menisci are composed of hyaline cartilage.
   c) The meniscus is an avascular structure.
   d) The medial and lateral menisci have equal mobility.
   e) The lateral and medial menisci are symmetric in shape and size.

The correct answer is (**a**). Each medial and lateral meniscus typically contains anterior and posterior root insertions attaching to the central tibial plateau. These anchors serve as primary stabilizers to maintain meniscal position and normal biomechanical function. The menisci are composed of fibrocartilage with circumferential and radially oriented collagen bundles that assist with hoop stress displacement.

The adult meniscus is separated into a peripheral one-third red zone or vascular zone and a central two-thirds white zone or avascular zone. Tears occurring within the red zone are more apt to spontaneously heal given the superimposed vascularity. The medial meniscus is less mobile because of its peripheral attachments to the deep fibers of the medial collateral ligament. The lateral meniscus is more symmetric and C-shaped in appearance, while the medial meniscus is crescentic in shape. The posterior horn medial meniscus is always larger in size than the anterior horn.

■ Case 23

1. Which of the following statements is false?
   a) The radial and ulnar collateral ligaments serve as the primary static stabilizers of the thumb metacarpal phalangeal (MCP) joint.
   b) A volar plate is not present at the thumb MCP joint.
   c) Tears of the ulnar collateral ligament at the thumb MCP joint are the most common injuries of the hand resulting from valgus stress.
   d) Any subluxation of the thumb MCP joint should be considered pathologic.
   e) Both b and d are false.

The correct answer is (**e**). The radial and ulnar collateral ligaments serve as the primary stabilizers of the thumb MCP joint and are intimately associated with the volar plate which is positioned over the volar surface of this joint. Ulnar collateral ligament injuries of the thumb MCP joint are reported to be the most common hand-related injury typically occurring from a valgus related force. Caution must be exercised when interpreting stress radiographs of the thumb MCP joint, as valgus angulation may normally range between 20 and 30 degrees depending on the degree of flexion.

2. Which of the following is true regarding the "yo-yo on a string" sign?
   a) The proximally retracted and rounded ulnar collateral ligament represents the yo-yo, and the string is represented by the adductor pollicis aponeurosis.
   b) The volar plate represents the string, and the retracted ulnar collateral ligament represents the yo-yo.
   c) This sign is best displayed on axial images through the thumb MCP joint.
   d) The proximally retracted and rounded ulnar collateral ligament represents the yo-yo, and the string is represented by the abductor pollicis tendon.
   e) None of the above is true.

The correct answer is (**a**). The Stener lesion has been described as a "yo-yo on a string." The thin adductor pollicis aponeurosis represents the string, which is positioned deep and just distal to the ruptured, proximally retracted, and rounded ulnar collateral ligament, or yo-yo.

■ Case 24

1. Regarding acromioclavicular (AC) joint separations, which of the following is false?
   a) Grades 1 and 2 separations are not detectable on radiography.
   b) Grade 4 injury involves a grade 3 injury with posterior displacement of the distal clavicle.
   c) A grade 5 AC joint injury is considered a severe grade 3 injury with 100 to 300% superior displacement of the clavicle relative to the acromion which may impinge into the trapezius musculature.
   d) All of the above are true.

The correct answer is (**a**). Grade 1 AC joint separation involves a capsular sprain with no abnormalities detected on radiography. A grade 2 AC joint injury involves disruption of the AC ligaments with minimal widening of the AC joint detected on radiographs. A grade 4 AC joint injury includes all components of a grade 3 injury in addition to posterior displacement of the clavicle relative to the acromion. A grade 5 AC joint injury represents a severe grade 3 injury with > 100% superior distraction of the clavicle relative to the acromion.

2. Components of the coracoclavicular ligament include which of the following?
   a) Coracohumeral ligament
   b) Conoid ligament
   c) Trapezoid ligament
   d) Answers b and c
   e) All of the above

The correct answer is (**d**). The coracoclavicular ligament is a primary stabilizer of the AC joint, preventing superior displacement of the clavicle. This complex consists of the conoid and trapezoid ligaments, which conform to the shape of the letter V.

■ Case 25

1. Which of the following statements is true regarding the hamstrings?
   a) The hamstring spans two joints, increasing susceptibility to injury.
   b) Proximal hamstring tendon avulsion may occur with severe stretching.
   c) Patients with hamstring tendon ruptures frequently complain of sciatic nerve symptoms given the proximity of the hamstring tendon to the sciatic nerve.
   d) All of the above statements are true.

The correct answer is (**d**). The hamstring musculature spans the hip and knee joint, increasing susceptibility to tearing/rupture. An additional mechanism for rupture of the proximal hamstring tendon complex is seen with forceful stretching with the hip flexed and the knee extended. Given the proximity of the sciatic nerve to the proximal hamstring tendon complex, focal inflammation from tendon rupture may cause sciatic nerve symptoms.

2. Regarding hamstring tendon anatomy, all of the following are true except...
   a) The muscle belly of the semitendinosus is the most cephalad of the hamstring muscle groups.
   b) The semitendinosus inserts distally along the anterior and medial proximal tibia.
   c) The semimembranosus has multiple insertion sites distally along the tibia.
   d) The biceps femoris has a short head which arises from the mid-diaphysis of the femur laterally.
   e) The primary distal biceps femoris insertion is on the lateral tibial metaphysis.

The correct answer is (**e**). The muscle belly of the semitendinosus is the most proximal of the hamstring musculature. The semitendinosus inserts distally along the anteromedial proximal tibia adjacent to the gracilis and sartorius to form the pes anserine tendons. The semimembranosus has multiple distal tibial tendinous insertions. The biceps femoris short-head muscle belly arises from the proximal femur laterally. The distal biceps femoris tendon primary insertion is upon the fibular head, with co-dominant slips attaching to the proximal lateral tibial metaphysis.

■ Case 26

1. MRI findings associated with adhesive capsulitis include which of the following?
   a) Anterior capsular stripping and a joint effusion
   b) Contrast enhancement of the inferior glenohumeral ligament and rotator interval structures
   c) A high-riding humeral head
   d) Medial subluxation of the biceps tendon

The correct answer is (**b**). MRI findings suggesting adhesive capsulitis include soft tissue thickening, edema, and enhancement of the rotator interval. The rotator interval is composed of the coracohumeral ligament and the superior glenohumeral ligament and is traversed by the biceps tendon. Capsular and inferior glenohumeral ligament edema and enhancement are also common features of adhesive capsulitis.

2. Which of the following structures borders the rotator interval?
   a) The anterior supraspinatus tendon
   b) The superior subscapularis tendon
   c) The acromion process
   d) All of the above
   e) Answers a and b

The correct answer is (**e**). The rotator interval is bordered by the supraspinatus muscle and tendon posteriorly and superiorly and the subscapularis muscle and tendon anteriorly and inferiorly. The acromion process does not border the rotator interval.

■ Case 27

1. Secondary signs of a posterior tibialis tendon tear include which of the following?
   a) Medial uncoverage of the talar head
   b) Hindfoot valgus deformity
   c) Talar beaking
   d) All of the above
   e) Both a and b

The correct answer is (**e**). Several anatomic changes may be observed with posterior tibialis tendon tearing. Medial uncoverage of the talar head may result secondary to unopposed pull of the midfoot and forefoot from the peroneus brevis. An additional observation is hindfoot or heel valgus angulation best displayed on coronal MR images comparing lines along the long axes of the calcaneus and the tibia. An additional finding is plantar flexion of the talus or midfoot collapse. This is best displayed on a lateral weightbearing radiograph of the foot. A line is drawn bisecting the longitudinal axis of the talus. This line should normally be in alignment with the longitudinal axis of the first metatarsal. With midfoot collapse, this line through the talus will lie inferior to the long axis of the metatarsals, indicating posterior tibialis tendon dysfunction.

2. The most common location for posterior tibialis tendon tears occurs at:
   a) The navicular insertion
   b) The perimalleolar region
   c) At the level of the distal tibial metaphysis
   d) No distinct level is particularly prone to tearing

The correct answer is (**b**). The most common location of posterior tibialis tendon disorders is the peri-malleolar region. This is believed to be related to the excess friction from the 90-degree turn made by the tendon at this site. A second location in which tears occur is more distally at the navicular insertion. This particular site is prone to tearing in athletic individuals or patients with inflammatory arthropathies.

■ Case 28

1. All of the following are typical pulmonary causes of hypertrophic osteoarthropathy except…
   a) Tumors of the pleura and mediastinum
   b) Lung abscess
   c) Bronchiectasis
   d) Hamartoma
   e) Empyema

The correct answer is (**d**). Pulmonary causes of hypertrophic osteoarthropathy include pulmonary infections, cystic fibrosis, cardiac shunts, and solitary fibrous tumor of the pleura/mediastinum/lung parenchyma. Pulmonary hamartoma has not been described as a cause of hypertrophic osteoarthropathy.

2. Systemic causes of hypertrophic osteoarthropathy include which of the following?
   a) Thyroid acropachy
   b) Rheumatoid arthritis
   c) Hyperparathyroidism/renal osteodystrophy
   d) All of the above
   e) Answers a and c

The correct answer is (**e**). Thyroid acropachy is a complication related to autoimmune thyroid disease producing symmetric spiculated periosteal reaction involving the mid-diaphyses of the tubular bones of the hands and feet. Secondary hyperparathyroidism is an additional cause of diffuse periosteal reaction related to parathyroid hormone stimulation of osteoblasts, resulting in linear periosteal new bone formation paralleling the cortical surface of the long bones of the upper and lower extremities. A relationship between hypertrophic osteoarthropathy and rheumatoid arthritis has not been established.

■ Case 29

1. Conditions that typically affect the first extensor compartment tendons include which of the following?
   a) Rheumatoid arthritis
   b) Calcium pyrophosphate dihydrate disease (CPPD) arthropathy
   c) Intersection syndrome
   d) Both a and c
   e) Both b and c

The correct answer is (**d**). Rheumatoid arthritis is a seropositive inflammatory arthropathy known for causing diffuse tenosynovitis. CPPD arthropathy represents a crystalline arthropathy not typically known for causing extensive tenosynovitis. Intersection syndrome represents a frictional tenosynovitis at the intersection of the first and second extensor tendon compartments ~4 to 6 cm proximal to the wrist joint.

2. Which of the following statements is true regarding the first extensor tendon compartment?
   a) Anatomic variation exists regarding the anatomy of the first extensor compartment, which is believed to contribute to de Quervain's tenosynovitis.
   b) The flexor retinaculum contributes to the roof of the first extensor tendon compartment.
   c) The EPB attaches to the distal phalanx of the thumb.
   d) The abductor pollicis longus (APL) attaches to the base of the proximal phalanx of the thumb.

The correct answer is (**a**). Studies have revealed further compartmentalization of the first extensor compartment with intervening septae bisecting the APL tendon possibly contributing to de Quervain's tenosynovitis. The extensor retinaculum contributes to the roof of the first extensor tendon compartment. The APL attaches to the dorsal base of the thumb metacarpal, whereas the EPB attaches to the base of the proximal phalanx of the thumb.

■ Case 30

1. Regarding the anatomy of the subtalar joint, which of the following statements is true?
   a) This joint consists of posterior, middle, and anterior articulating facets.
   b) The middle facet is the most lateral of all the articular facets.
   c) The sustentaculum talus is a component of the posterior facet.
   d) The largest of the articular facets is the anterior facet.

The correct answer is (**a**). The subtalar joint is composed of anterior, middle, and posterior facets. The smallest of these facets is the anterior facet and the largest and most lateral is the posterior facet. The sustentaculum talus of the calcaneus contains the middle facet calcaneal articular surface.

2. Regarding the various types of tarsal coalitions, which of the following statements is false?
   a) Synchondroses, syndesmoses, or synostoses are terms used to describe the various types of coalitions.
   b) The frequency of talocalcaneal and calcaneonavicular coalitions is approximately the same.
   c) MRI more frequently demonstrates bone marrow edema in the setting of osseous coalitions.
   d) Tarsal coalitions may be intra- or extra-articular.

The correct answer is (**c**). Tarsal coalition composed of cartilage represents a synchondrosis, fibrous coalition is referred to as a syndesmosis, and an osseous coalition is synonymous with a synostosis. Talocalcaneal and calcaneonavicular coalitions occur with similar frequency. Intra- and extra-articular tarsal coalitions have been described. The most commonly observed extra-articular coalition lies between the posterior margin of the susten-taculum talus and the posterior medial process of the talus posterior to the middle facet. MR findings of bone marrow edema frequently coexist with fibrous and cartilaginous coalitions related to the limited motion and secondary stress changes not typically seen with fixed complete osseous coalitions.

■ **Case 31**

1. Regarding an anterior cruciate ligament (ACL) ganglion cyst, which of the following statements is true?
    a) These cysts contain a synovial lining.
    b) Adjacent bony cystic changes are identical in histopathology to the ACL ganglion cysts.
    c) These cysts are typically seen along the distal ACL.
    d) All of the above are false.

The correct answer is (**b**). ACL ganglion cysts do not have a true synovial lining distinguishing them from synovial cysts. The composition of these cysts is mucoid degenera-tion. This is identical in composition to the adjacent cystic osseous changes which are likely caused by extrinsic ero-sion. ACL cysts may be observed along the entire length of the ligament.

2. Regarding cruciate ligament mucoid degeneration, which of the following is true?
    a) May occur in both the ACL and PCL
    b) Is not a bilateral process
    c) Is associated with a narrow intercondylar notch
    d) Is more common in females

The correct answer is (**a**). Cruciate mucoid degeneration has been reported in both the ACL and PCL, occurring more frequently in the ACL. Bilateral cruciate ligament involve-ment has also been observed, lending credence to a degen-erative senescent etiology. A narrowed intercondylar notch has been found to have no association with this condition. No gender predilection has been reported to date.

■ **Case 32**

1. Which of the following statements is true concerning joint aspiration in the setting of infected arthroplasty components?
    a) The absence of joint fluid excludes infection.
    b) Discontinuation of antibiotics is recommended to optimize the detection of infection.
    c) Aspirated synovial fluid cultures demonstrating no growth excludes infection.
    d) Cell count and differential of aspirated joint fluid offers minimal assistance with the diagnosis of infection.

The correct answer is (**b**). Although many joints with infected arthroplasty components may contain fluid, it is not uncommon for these articulations to contain synovitis/synovial thickening with minimal to no fluid. The diagnostic sensitivity for infection after joint aspiration is 75 to 100%, the specificity is 96 to 100%, and the accuracy is 90 to 100%. Patients must have discontinued antibiotic therapy for at least 4 weeks to achieve these optimal results. Analysis of aspirated fluid should also include cell count and differ-ential to help assist with the diagnosis. An abundance of neutrophils would be expected in the setting of infection.

2. Expected nuclear medicine findings in the setting of hardware infection include which of the following?
    a) Negative three-phase bone scan
    b) Positive uptake on the second phase of a three-phase bone scan
    c) Positive uptake on all phases of the three-phase bone scan with positive uptake on a tagged white blood cell scan
    d) Positive uptake on the delayed phase of the three-phase bone scan with negative uptake on a tagged white blood cell scan

The correct answer is (**c**). Nuclear medicine examinations and techniques (labeled white blood cell scans, three-phase bone scans) may show a wide range of results. Increased or positive uptake on all three phases of a three-phase bone scan may be seen with hardware infection. Likewise, a high negative predictive value is seen with a negative three-phase bone scan. Labeled white blood cell imaging is well suited to determine the presence of an infected prosthesis. Neutrophils will accumulate in the in-fected joint, allowing for increased white blood cell uptake. When combined with bone marrow imaging, tagged white blood cell imaging is ~90% accurate.

■ **Case 33**

1. Lisfranc ligamentous complex is composed of:
    a) A single and structurally weak dorsal bundle which accounts for frequent dorsal metatarsal subluxation
    b) A single bundle running from the medial cuneiform to the second metatarsal base
    c) Three separate bundles running from the medial cuneiform to the second and third metatarsal bases
    d) A joint capsule with a synovial lining
    e) None of the above

The correct answer is (**c**). The Lisfranc ligament com-plex is composed of three separate obliquely oriented ligaments—the dorsal, plantar, and common/interosseous ligaments. The common interosseous and dorsal ligaments run from the medial cuneiform to the second metatarsal base. The plantar ligament runs from the medial cuneiform with variable insertions along the plantar bases of the second and third metatarsals. The dorsal band is the weakest of the ligamentous structures and may account for the frequent dorsal metatarsal base subluxation seen with Lisfranc injuries.

2. The Lisfranc joint provides:
   a) Maintenance of the transverse arch of the foot
   b) Stabilization to the tarsometatarsal (TMT) joints
   c) Stabilization between the bases of the first and second metatarsals, which are void of an intermetatarsal ligament
   d) All of the above are true

The correct answer is (**d**). Lisfranc joint refers to the articulation involving the first and second metatarsals and the medial and intermediate cuneiforms. This articulation assists with maintenance of the transverse arch of the foot and stabilization of the TMT junction. Additionally, no interosseous ligament lies between the bases of the first and second metatarsals. Therefore, the Lisfranc ligament complex provides stabilization at this interval.

■ **Case 34**

1. Regarding chondroblastomas, which of the following is true?
   a) Metaphyseal involvement with a cartilage lesion excludes chondroblastoma.
   b) Periosteal reaction is frequently seen with these lesions.
   c) This lesion is equally distributed between males and females.
   d) Chondroblastoma has not been reported in the patella.
   e) The most common location for chondroblastoma in the foot and ankle is the cuneiforms.

The correct answer is (**b**). A variable degree of metaphyseal extension is typical for chondroblastoma with the bulk of the tumor localized to the epiphysis. Mature periosteal reaction is present in the majority of chondroblastomas, typically seen in the metaphysis adjacent to the epiphyseal lesion. Chondroblastoma has a male-to-female ratio of nearly 3:1. Chondroblastoma represents ~15% of all reported lesions within the patella. The foot and ankle represents the second most common site for chondroblastoma, after the long bones. In this region, chondroblastoma most commonly involves the talus and calcaneus.

2. Decreased T1 and T2 signal on MR imaging of chondroblastoma is related to which of the following?
   a) Abundant collagen and fibrous tissue superimposed upon chronic blood products
   b) Abundant osseous matrix
   c) Immature chondroid matrix with hypercellular chondroblasts, calcifications, and hemosiderin
   d) Mature chondroid matrix superimposed upon chronic blood products

The correct answer is (**c**). Approximately 60% of chondroblastomas display intermediate to decreased T1 and T2 signal related to immature chondroid matrix and an abundance of chondroblasts with superimposed chondroid calcifications and hemosiderin.

■ **Case 35**

1. Which of the following describes the normal ultrasound appearance of the biceps tendon?
   a) Contains a prominent longitudinal sonolucent cleft
   b) Proximal fusiform enlargement with surrounding sonolucent fluid
   c) Hyperechoic, uniform in size, and fibrillar
   d) None of the above

The correct answer is (**c**). The biceps tendon should normally appear linear, uniform in size, hyperechoic, and fibrillar. These findings are related to intact tightly bound collagen fibers. Trace physiologic fluid may lie posterior to the tendon. Circumferential sonolucent fluid suggests tenosynovitis. A split tear of the biceps tendon manifests with a longitudinally oriented hypoechoic/sonolucent cleft.

2. The ideal technique for performing an ultrasound of the biceps tendon includes which of the following?
   a) The patient's arm should be flexed and placed above the head.
   b) The patient's palm should be facing down and the transducer should be aligned in the transverse and longitudinal planes of the tendon.
   c) The patient's palm should be facing up and the transducer should be aligned in the transverse and longitudinal planes of the tendon.
   d) The patient's arm should be placed behind the back with the dorsum of the wrist placed against the back.

The correct answer is (**c**). Ideal positioning for exposure and evaluation of the biceps tendon requires the patient's palm facing up on the lap, resulting in external rotation of the shoulder. This positions the biceps sulcus over the anterior aspect of the shoulder. The transducer should be positioned in both the axial and longitudinal planes of the biceps tendon, allowing for optimal evaluation along its entire course.

■ **Case 36**

1. Which of the following lesions typically does not exhibit coexisting secondary aneurysmal bone cyst (ABC) features?
   a) Giant cell tumor of the bone
   b) Telangiectatic osteosarcoma
   c) Osteoid osteoma
   d) Chondroblastoma
   e) Osteoblastoma

The correct answer is (**c**). Up to 30% of diagnosed ABCs may be secondary to a superimposed hemorrhage within a solid bony lesion. These secondary aneurysmal bone cyst changes are well described in fibrous dysplasia, osteoblastoma, giant cell tumor of the bone, chondroblastoma, telangiectatic osteosarcoma, and nonossifying fibromas. Osteoid osteoma does not exhibit these secondary changes.

2. Which of the following statements is false regarding ABCs?
    a) Fluid–fluid levels relate to layering blood-filled locules surrounded by connective tissue and giant cells.
    b) Solid and soft tissue variants exist.
    c) These lesions have a moderate malignant potential.
    d) All of the above statements are false.

The correct answer is (**c**). The typical primary ABC consists of multiple loculated blood-filled spaces accounting for the fluid–fluid levels. There are intervening septae composed of connective tissue with giant cells. Solid, soft tissue, and periosteal variants of ABCs have been described, although they are much less common than the intramedullary form. Malignant degeneration is not typically seen.

■ **Case 37**
··

1. Which of the following statements is false?
    a) The least common plica is the lateral plica.
    b) Plicae, when present, are most often asymptomatic.
    c) The infrapatellar plica courses adjacent to the PCL.
    d) Direct or indirect trauma to plicae is believed to be a causative factor for plica syndrome.

The correct answer is (**c**). Superior, inferior, and medial plicae most commonly exist and are usually asymptomatic. Less than 1% of patients will have a lateral plica. The superior and inferior plicae occur with equal frequency. Second in frequency is the medial plica. The infrapatellar plica, or ligamentum mucosum, parallels the ACL anteriorly originating from the intercondylar notch of the femur extending anteriorly to insert within the infrapatellar fat or upon the inferior pole of the patella. Plica syndrome typically results from trauma related to a twisting injury.

2. Which of the following statements is true regarding the origin of synovial plicae?
    a) Synovial plicae originate from cartilage rests adjacent to the patella, femur, or tibial articular surfaces.
    b) Synovial plicae is a misnomer because these structures represent vestigial accessory ligaments.
    c) Synovial plicae represent embryologic septal remnants of synovium.
    d) Synovial plicae originate as a result of childhood and adolescent microtrauma.

The correct answer is (**c**). Embryologically, the knee joint is separated into three synovial compartments. There is subsequent near-complete involution of these compartments. The remaining synovial remnants are referred to as plicae. These embryologic remnants have no cartilage or ligamentous homolog.

■ **Case 38**
··

1. The MRI demonstration of a "J" sign of a HAGL refers to the following:
    a) Posttraumatic edema pattern present within the axillary soft tissues
    b) The labral tear pattern
    c) The alignment pattern of the glenohumeral joint
    d) The appearance of the inferior glenohumeral ligament on coronal oblique images

The correct answer is (**d**). The "J" sign indicates humeral avulsion of the glenohumeral ligament. The normal anatomic configuration of the inferior glenohumeral ligament is oriented in the shape of a "U" on coronal MR imaging. This ligament attaches to the glenoid labrum medially and the surgical neck of the humerus laterally. Avulsion of the humeral attachment of this ligament transforms the U shape to a J shape.

2. Which of the following describes the primary function of the inferior glenohumeral ligament?
    a) The main anterior dynamic stabilizer of the shoulder when the arm is abducted, preventing anterior dislocation during external rotation
    b) The main anterior static stabilizer of the shoulder when the arm is abducted, preventing anterior dislocation during external rotation
    c) The main static stabilizer of the shoulder joint when the arm is adducted, preventing superior subluxation
    d) The main dynamic stabilizer of the shoulder joint when the arm is adducted, preventing superior subluxation

The correct answer is (**b**). The inferior glenohumeral ligament is a hammocklike structure containing thickened anterior and posterior bands. The anterior band is believed to represent the major static stabilizer of the glenohumeral joint upon abduction and external rotation, preventing anterior dislocation. Other static restraining structures include the remaining glenohumeral ligaments, the coracohumeral ligament, the glenoid labrum, and the glenohumeral joint. Dynamic stabilizers include the rotator cuff and biceps tendons.

■ Case 39

1. Regarding patellar cartilage, which of the following statements is true?
   a) The patellar cartilage is composed of a combination of fibrocartilage and hyaline cartilage.
   b) The patellar cartilage is composed of hyaline cartilage and is the thickest of all articular cartilage surfaces in the human body.
   c) The patella is a common site for cartilage harvest.
   d) Patellar articular cartilage defects may regenerate hyaline cartilage.

The correct answer is (**b**). The patellar articular cartilage is composed of hyaline cartilage and represents the thickest articular cartilage in humans. The trochlear articular cartilage is a common site for cartilage graft harvest. Patellar cartilage defects do not have the ability to regenerate hyaline cartilage. Instead, fibrocartilage regrowth occurs.

2. Which of the following is believed to represent the etiology of the dorsal defect of the patella (DDP)?
   a) A genetic segmentation anomaly
   b) Mechanical traction and/or epiphyseal developmental alteration
   c) A vascular phenomenon
   d) Cartilage hydration anomaly

The correct answer is (**b**). The proposed etiology for the DDP is unclear, with working hypotheses suggesting alteration of the normal epiphyseal formation of the patella and/or a mechanical traction abnormality along the lateral patellar facet. Some studies have suggested the DDP may exist as part of a continuum leading to a bipartite patella.

■ Case 40

1. Which of the following statements is false?
   a) The peak incidence of giant cell tumor (GCT) is in patients between 25 and 50 years of age.
   b) Secondary aneurysmal bone cyst may occur in up to 14% of GCTs.
   c) In addition to curettage and cementation, the monoclonal antibody denosumab has been used to prevent recurrence.
   d) GCT is common in the spine.

The correct answer is (**d**). The peak incidence of GCT occurs between 25 and 50 years of age with the prevalence of patients presenting during the third decade. Secondary aneurysmal bone cyst components containing fluid–fluid levels may be seen in ~14% of all GCTs, necessitating biopsy directed at the solid tissue for accurate diagnosis. Use of the monoclonal antibody denosumab has resulted in a dramatic treatment response. This drug inhibits the osteoclastic effects of this lesion. GCTs are relatively uncommon in the spine and, when present, typically involve the vertebral body.

2. Features of GCT recurrence include:
   a) Lucent bony changes along the margins of curettage
   b) Sclerosis along the margins of curettage
   c) Development of a soft tissue mass along the bony margins of resection
   d) All of the above
   e) Both a and c

The correct answer is (**e**). Bone and soft tissue tumor recurrence may occur following GCT resection and is best identified by comparing follow-up images with the initial baseline postoperative imaging. Bony recurrence requires close inspection of follow-up radiographs for development of any new lucency at the cementation–bone interface. CT will allow for optimal evaluation of this osteolysis, whereas MR imaging enables better detection of a soft tissue mass recurring within the operative bed.

■ Case 41

1. Regarding ganglion cysts, which of the following is true?
   a) May cause neurologic symptoms
   b) More common in men
   c) Most commonly affect the left hand
   d) Radiographs are sufficient for complete evaluation
   e) Typically contain calcifications

The correct answer is (**a**). Ganglion cysts may cause neurologic symptoms, particularly if in proximity to the triquetral pisiform articulation where the cyst causes mass effect on the ulnar nerve. There is a 2:1 female predominance of ganglion cysts. Both hands are equally affected with ganglion cysts. Radiographs are typically not sufficient for complete characterization, with US serving as the simplest and least expensive imaging modality for further assessment. Ganglion cysts do not contain calcifications. If calcifications are present, consider an alternative diagnosis.

2. Ganglion cysts are typically located in all of the following locations within the hand and wrist except...
   a) Carpal tunnel floor
   b) Flexor and extensor tendons
   c) Annular pulleys of the fingers
   d) Interosseous and lumbrical musculature
   e) Nailbed of the finger

The correct answer is (**d**). Carpal tunnel syndrome related to compressive neuropathy of the median nerve secondary to a carpal tunnel floor ganglion cyst may occur, albeit rarely. Ganglion cysts may frequently be seen adjacent to flexor and extensor tendons, particularly the flexor carpi radialis tendon. Ganglion cysts may arise from the volar flexor surface of the fingers typically associated with the annular pulleys A1 or A2. Ganglion cyst formation also may occur along the external surface of the extensor tendon insertion onto the distal phalanx with extension into the nailbed. Ganglion cysts originating from the musculature of the hand are not typical and an alternative diagnosis should be considered.

■ Case 42

1. Which of the following statements is true regarding the middle third lateral capsular ligament?
   a) Cordlike ligament running from the distal femur to the tibial insertion of the iliotibial band or Gerdy's tubercle
   b) Thin ligament running from the lateral femoral epicondyle inserting posterior to the fibular collateral ligament
   c) Thin ligament extending from the lateral femoral epicondyle to the proximal tibia inserting posterior to Gerdy's tubercle
   d) Cordlike structure running adjacent to the iliotibial band
   e) Thin ligament running from the distal lateral femur inseparable from the lateral patellofemoral retinaculum

The correct answer is (c). The middle third lateral capsular ligament is described as a sheetlike thin ligament along the lateral knee joint line. This ligament extends from the lateral femoral epicondyle and inserts onto the body of the lateral meniscus and proximal tibia. This structure courses anterior to the fibular collateral ligament and inserts immediately distal to the lateral tibial plateau and posterior to Gerdy's tubercle. This ligament frequently serves as the site of insertion for the Segond fracture fragment. The posterior iliotibial band less frequently attaches to this fragment. Of note, the term anterior lateral ligament may be used synonymously with middle third lateral capsular ligament.

2. In addition to ACL tears, which of the following injuries may also be seen with the Segond fracture?
   a) Meniscal tears, posterior lateral corner injuries
   b) Patellofemoral retinacular and gastrocnemius injuries
   c) Patellar chondral defects
   d) Adductor magnus avulsions

The correct answer is (a). The typical mechanism of injury for a Segond fracture is internal rotation with varus stress applied to the knee, placing force on the lateral joint capsule. As a result, injury to the posterior lateral corner ligamentous and tendinous structures occurs. Additionally, contusions and/or fractures to the lateral tibial plateau, lateral femoral condyle contusions, and medial/lateral meniscal tearing are seen.

■ Case 43

1. Regarding osteopoikilosis, which of the following statements is false?
   a) A genetic condition
   b) More commonly seen in females
   c) Considered a disorder of membranous bone formation
   d) Referred to as the "spotted bone disease"
   e) Falls into a class of disorders that also includes osteopathia striatum and melorheostosis

The correct answer is (c). Osteopoikilosis displays an autosomal-dominant inheritance pattern with equal frequency in males and females. An alternative name for this disease is "spotted bone disease" given its appearance on radiographs. This is considered a sclerosing bony dystrophy or dysplasia. Hereditary forms of bony dysplasias include osteopetrosis, pyknodysostosis, and osteopathia striata, among others. Nonhereditary dysplasias include melorheostosis. Osteopoikilosis is a disorder of enchondral ossification involving the secondary spongiosa.

2. All of the following may be associated with sclerotic skeletal changes except…
   a) Paget's disease
   b) Enostosis
   c) Prostate cancer
   d) Rheumatoid arthritis
   e) Pyknodysostosis

The correct answer is (d). Paget's disease is a disorder of bony remodeling consisting of a blastic and lytic phase. An enostosis is also referred to as a bone island represented by a solitary and dense focus of compact bone formation. Blastic metastases in the human skeleton are commonly seen with prostate cancer. Pyknodysostosis is a hereditary bony dysplasia characterized by skeletal osteosclerosis and short stature. Rheumatoid arthritis is a symmetric and deforming erosive arthropathy demonstrating periarticular osteopenia without sclerotic skeletal changes.

■ Case 44

1. Regarding Morton's neuromas, which of the following statements is true?
   a) These lesions are symptomatic only in the presence of intermetatarsal bursal fluid.
   b) Neuromas > 2 mm in size tend to be more symptomatic.
   c) Morton's neuromas are described in both men and women.
   d) Administration of gadolinium offers no advantage in detection on MRI.

The correct answer is (**c**). Distention of the intermetatarsal bursae is commonly seen in both symptomatic and asymptomatic patients with a Morton's neuroma. Neuromas > 5 mm in size tend to be more symptomatic. These lesions are described in both males and females. The conspicuity of Morton's neuroma is increased with the administration of gadolinium on MR imaging.

2. Morton's neuroma is most commonly seen in the second and third intermetatarsal spaces as a result of which one of the following?
   a) The second and third intermetatarsal spaces are larger in size compared with the remaining intermetatarsal spaces.
   b) A true bursa exists at these levels.
   c) The second and third intermetatarsal spaces are smaller in size compared with the remaining intermetatarsal spaces.
   d) Maximum force occurs through these intermetatarsal spaces with forefoot loading.

The correct answer is (**c**). The Morton's neuroma most frequently occurs in the second and third intermetatarsal spaces. This is related to the narrow interval between these metatarsal heads resulting in increased friction upon the digital plantar nerves with forefoot loading. The third intermetatarsal space serves as the most common site for this lesion followed in frequency by the second intermetatarsal space.

■ **Case 45**

1. Complications of Paget's disease include all of the following except…
   a) Insufficiency fractures
   b) Multiple sclerosis
   c) Transformation to osteosarcoma
   d) Giant cell tumor
   e) Neurologic entrapment

The correct answer is (**b**). Complications of Paget's disease include fracture and bowing deformities secondary to an imbalance between osteoclastic and osteoblastic activity. An underlying viral infection has been implicated in this disease process. Neoplastic transformation with this disease is not typical and may include degeneration into osteosarcoma, seen in ~5 to 10% of cases. Giant cell tumor formation is extremely uncommon and may occur in the skull and facial bones. Neurologic entrapment is most often reported in the skull secondary to overgrowth of the inner table, causing cranial nerve entrapment and neurosensory disturbances. Multiple sclerosis has no association with Paget's disease.

2. Osteoporosis circumscripta refers to which of the following?
   a) The radiographic appearance of the mixed phase of Paget's within the skull
   b) The silent and asymptomatic or blastic phase of Paget's disease within the skull
   c) Localized osteopenia resulting from a pagetic insufficiency fracture
   d) The lytic phase of this disease within the skull

The correct answer is (**d**). The lytic phase of Paget's disease within the skull results in an appearance known as osteoporosis circumscripta. This is manifested radiographically by circumscribed geographic osteolysis typically involving the frontal and occipital bones. Radionuclide uptake will be confined to the margins of the affected skull.

■ **Case 46**

1. Common locations for the Morel–Lavallee lesion (MLL) include the following:
   a) Knee, gluteal region, lumbar spine
   b) Scalp and forefoot
   c) Hand and wrist
   d) Abdomen and chest wall

The correct answer is (**a**). Although the most common location for the MLL is adjacent to the greater trochanter, this lesion has been reported adjacent to the knee, gluteus musculature, and lumbar spine. Much less commonly reported locations are adjacent to the scalp, scapula, shoulder, ankle, and hand.

2. Which of the following allows distinction of prepatellar bursitis from MLL?
   a) Bursitis will typically exhibit synovial thickening.
   b) MLL may extend beyond the confines of the bursa.
   c) Bursitis will not contain blood products.
   d) MLL will resolve over time.

The correct answer is (**b**). The fluid collection associated with MLL may extend beyond the typical anatomic confines of the prepatellar bursa in craniocaudal and medial lateral dimensions. Prepatellar bursitis may or may not demonstrate synovial thickening and its absence is not a reliable discriminator from MLL. Hemorrhagic prepatellar bursitis may be seen with repetitive microtrauma or severe direct trauma. Most cases of prepatellar bursitis will improve or resolve over time and respond to steroid injection. MLL lesions typically will not resolve in time. MLL adjacent to the patella is recognized in many contact sports, such as wrestling and football.

■ Case 47

1. Proper positioning of the femoral tunnel with anterior cruciate ligament (ACL) reconstruction optimizes which of the following functions?
   a) Coronal balance
   b) Lateral joint line stability
   c) Graft tension
   d) Patellofemoral tracking

The correct answer is (**c**). Femoral tunnel positioning allows constant tensioning on the ACL graft throughout flexion and extension. The femoral tunnel should be aligned at the intersection of the physeal scar of the distal femur and the posterior intercondylar roof. A malpositioned and anteriorly located femoral tunnel elongates the ACL graft causing instability.

2. Which of the following statements is true regarding the normal MRI appearance of an ACL graft?
   a) Signal changes should normalize ~1 year following graft placement.
   b) Signal increase should be present indefinitely.
   c) Absence of signal intensity should be present 8 weeks following surgery.
   d) Any signal change after 6 months should be considered abnormal.

The correct answer is (**a**). When interpreting MRI of the postoperative ACL graft, it is important to realize that graft synovialization and vascularization may occur for up to 1 to 2 years following surgery. On MR imaging, these changes are reflected by intermediate intrasubstance signal increase oriented along the longitudinal axis of the ACL graft.

These changes are most notable with multi-bundle hamstring grafts as opposed to single-bundle grafts such as the patellar tendon. Upon resolution of these changes, the ACL graft should demonstrate low MR signal intensity on all pulse sequences. Any subsequent deviation from these signal changes may represent pathology in the form of degeneration or partial tearing.

■ Case 48

1. Inherited conditions associated with an increased incidence of osteosarcoma include which of the following?
   a) Familial polyposis
   b) Hereditary retinoblastoma
   c) Li–Fraumeni syndrome
   d) Answers b and c
   e) All of the above

The correct answer is (**d**). Familial polyposis shows no increased risk for osteosarcoma. Li–Fraumeni syndrome represents a familial cancer syndrome with family members exhibiting multiple malignancies. These malignancies may include osteosarcoma, leukemia, brain/breast/soft tissue tumors, and adrenocortical tumors. This condition is likely related to a mutation in the *p53* gene. Hereditary retinoblastoma is associated with an increased risk of osteosarcomas. Additional genetic conditions predisposing to osteosarcoma include Rothmund–Thomson, Bloom's, and Werner's syndromes.

2. Which of the following conditions carry an increased risk of osteosarcoma?
   a) Paget's disease
   b) Prior radiation therapy
   c) Osteopathia striata
   d) Answers a and b
   e) All of the above

The correct answer is (**d**). Paget's disease is a disorder related to accelerated bone turnover leading to a slightly increased incidence of osteosarcoma. This transformation is typically seen in long-standing Paget's disease. Sarcomatous transformation is not necessarily related to the extent of skeletal involvement with Paget's. Osteosarcoma is the most frequent secondary malignancy following radiation therapy for solid tumors in childhood. Secondary osteosarcoma may arise within the first 12 to 16 years following radiation treatment. Approximately 3% of all osteosarcomas are attributed to prior irradiation. Osteopathia striata has no increased risk of malignancy.

■ Case 49

1. Other locations for glomus tumors include all of the following except...
   a) Gastrointestinal tract
   b) Soles of the feet
   c) Lungs
   d) Meninges
   e) Trachea

The correct answer is (**d**). Although the most common locations for glomus tumors include the fingers, palms, and soles of the feet, other reported locations include the gastrointestinal tract, lungs, trachea, and intraneural or intraosseous locations. The glomus tumor has not been described in the meninges.

2. Which of the following is suggestive of a malignant glomus tumor?
   a) Increased uptake on positron emission tomography (PET) scanning
   b) Lesion size > 1 cm
   c) Lesions that are positioned in a deep location
   d) Superficial lesions that markedly deform the skin surface

The correct answer is (**c**). Glomus tumors are typically benign. However, malignant glomus tumors should be suspected if they are positioned in a deep location and are > 2 cm in size. Benign glomus tumors may be fluorodeoxyglucose avid on PET imaging. It is not uncommon for superficial benign glomus tumors to alter the appearance of the skin surface.

■ Case 50

1. Which of the following represent functions of the extensor carpi ulnaris (ECU)?
    a) Radial deviation and abduction of the hand
    b) Extension and adduction of the hand
    c) Ulnar deviation of the hand
    d) Answers b and c
    e) All of the above

The correct answer is (**d**). The ECU inserts upon the dorsal base of the fifth metacarpal and is responsible for extension and adduction of the hand and assists with ulnar deviation.

2. Regarding the anatomy of the ECU, which of the following statements is true?
    a) It is composed of two separate muscle heads.
    b) A separate and distinct ligament secures this tendon at the ulnar styloid groove.
    c) Signal increase within the tendon at the ulnar styloid groove may be related to normal anatomy.
    d) All of the above are true.

The correct answer is (**d**). The ECU tendon arises from two separate muscle heads originating from the lateral epicondyle and mid-diaphysis of the ulna. The asymptomatic ECU tendon may normally exhibit mild intrasubstance signal increase at the ulnar styloid groove. This is related to interposed mucoid and collagen material present within a cleft formed by partially separated distal tendon slips at this site, termed the "pseudo-lesion." A ligament referred to as the subsheath overlies the ECU tendon at the distal groove and prevents tendon dislocation.

■ Case 51

1. MRI findings used for grading of tibial stress injuries include which of the following?
    a) Periosteal edema
    b) Bone marrow edema
    c) Intracortical signal abnormality
    d) Muscle edema and hypervascularity
    e) All of the above
    f) Answers a, b, and c

The correct answer is (**f**). The Fredericson classification scheme for grading tibial stress injuries is commonly used. Features of this grading system include periosteal edema

and cortical/bone marrow signal abnormalities. Fluid-sensitive MR imaging may demonstrate these findings. Muscle and vascular MR abnormalities are not included in this grading scheme.

2. Relatively common locations for stress injury in the healthy human skeleton include which of the following?
    a) Tarsal bones, metatarsals, fibula
    b) Sacrum, pubic rami, scapular neck
    c) Proximal medial tibial metaphysis, scapular neck
    d) Femoral head, medial femoral condyle

The correct answer is (**a**). The sacrum, pubic rami, scapular neck, proximal medial tibial metaphysis, femoral head, and medial femoral condyle all represent sites prone to insufficiency fractures in the osteoporotic skeleton. Commonly affected bony structures affiliated with stress injuries in the healthy human skeleton include the tarsal bones, metatarsals, and fibula, listed in decreasing order of frequency.

■ Case 52

1. Which of the following structures are important stabilizers for the posterior lateral corner of the knee?
    a) Iliotibial band, lateral patellofemoral retinaculum
    b) Lateral collateral ligament, biceps femoris tendon, popliteal fibular ligament
    c) Posterior oblique ligament, extensor mechanism
    d) Ligament of Humphrey, ligament of Wrisberg

The correct answer is (**b**). The posterior lateral aspect of the knee is stabilized functionally and anatomically by the lateral collateral ligament, biceps femoris tendon, popliteus muscle and tendon, popliteal meniscal ligament, popliteal fibular ligament, oblique popliteal and fabellofibular ligament's, and the lateral gastrocnemius muscle. The iliotibial band and lateral patellofemoral retinaculum lie over the anterior and lateral knee joint line offering minimal support for posterior lateral stability. The meniscal femoral ligaments primary role is to secure the lateral meniscus during the various phases of the knee motion. The posterior oblique ligament provides stability along the posterior and medial joint line. The extensor mechanism is primarily involved with patellofemoral stability.

2. Which of the following best describes the anatomy of the arcuate ligament?
    a) A fan-shaped musculotendinous unit arising from the posterior tibia with multiple insertions onto the lateral meniscus and fibula
    b) A cordlike structure easily detectable on MRI running from the fibular head to the lateral femoral condyle
    c) A Y-shaped structure representing thickening of the posterior lateral joint capsule
    d) An intersection of multiple tendons to include the plantaris and lateral head of the gastrocnemius

The correct answer is (c). The arcuate ligament is an important component of posterior lateral joint stability. This is a Y-shaped structure with the apex attaching to the fibular styloid process. The lateral limb of this ligament inserts into the posterior lateral joint capsule, whereas the medial limb extends superficial to the popliteus muscle inserting onto the oblique popliteal ligament. This structure is difficult to visualize on MRI and is best seen on sagittal images.

■ Case 53

1. Which of the following statements is correct regarding parosteal osteosarcoma?
    a) Represents a surface osteosarcoma having the best overall prognosis
    b) Frequently will demonstrate medullary canal invasion
    c) May be associated with prior radiation therapy
    d) Typically seen with Paget's disease

The correct answer is (a). Surface or juxtacortical osteosarcomas are composed of three variants including parosteal osteosarcoma, periosteal osteosarcoma, and high-grade surface osteosarcoma. Parosteal osteosarcoma represents the most common and least aggressive of these entities and may rarely invade the medullary canal. No definitive association with prior radiation therapy or Paget's disease exists with this subtype of osteosarcoma.

2. Regarding imaging of parosteal osteosarcoma, the reverse zonal phenomenon refers to which one of the following?
    a) Centripetal ossification with a central soft tissue mass
    b) Peripheral soft tissue mass with central osteoid mineralization
    c) Radiolucent cleavage plane between the ossified mass and cortex of a tubular bone
    d) Typical growth pattern seen with highly malignant bone-forming lesions

The correct answer is (b). The atypical growth pattern of central ossification with a peripheral soft tissue mass is characteristic for parosteal osteosarcoma. This reverse pattern of ossification is termed the *reverse zonal phenomenon* on imaging. This is in contradistinction to the zonal phenomenon described in the setting of myositis ossificans in which a benign reactive rim of mature bone encircles a central soft tissue mass or fluid.

■ Case 54

1. All of the following are potential causes of ulnar plus variance except...
    a) Chronic impaction fracture of the distal radial metaphysis
    b) Madelung's deformity
    c) Boxer's fracture
    d) Essex–Lopresti fracture

The correct answer is (c). Any congenital or posttraumatic condition resulting in shortening of the radius may cause ulnar plus variance. A distal radial malunion secondary to an impaction fracture may serve as a cause of ulnar plus variance. Premature ulnar fusion of the distal radial physis may lead to ulnar plus variance, as seen with a Madelung's deformity. The Essex–Lopresti fracture complex involves a comminuted impacted radial head fracture with disruption of the interosseous membrane and resultant radial foreshortening leading to ulnar plus variance. Boxer's fractures do not affect ulnar variance.

2. Which of the following statements regarding ulnar variance is false?
    a) Neutral or supinated positioning of the wrist and forearm allows the most accurate assessment of ulnar variance.
    b) Positioning of the distal ulna articular surface > 2 mm relative to the distal radial articular surface is referred to as ulnar plus variance.
    c) Pronated grip radiographs are most useful to assess ulnar plus variance.
    d) Conventional positioning of wrist radiographs may fail to display ulnar variance.

The correct answer is (a). The distal ulnar articular surface may normally lie between 1 and 2 mm proud to the distal radial articular surface. Ulnar variance > 2 mm distal to the radial surface is referred to as ulnar plus variance. Standard radiographic views of the wrist may fail to display the true variance of the distal ulna. The ideal positioning for assessing ulnar variance on radiographs is with forearm pronation in combination with a firm grip.

■ Case 55

1. Regarding the articular anatomy of the sacroiliac (SI) joints, which of the following statements is true?
    a) The superior 50% of the SI joints is a synovial-based articulation.
    b) Hyaline cartilage outlines both sides of the SI joint with erosive change and edema equally affecting both articular margins.
    c) The superior two thirds of the SI joints are fibrous in nature.
    d) Fibrocartilage outlines all margins of the SI joint.
    e) All of the above are true.

The correct answer is (**c**). The distal one third of the SI joint is synovial based. Thick hyaline cartilage coats the sacral side of the joint at this level. Thinner and less robust fibrocartilage lines the iliac side of this portion of the joint. It is these changes that account for the profuse bony structural alterations more commonly occurring along the iliac side of the SI joint when presented with infectious or inflammatory processes. The approximate proximal two thirds of the SI joint are bound by fibrous interosseous ligaments with this segment of the SI joint functioning as a syndesmosis.

2. Regarding MRI findings of sacroiliitis in patients with psoriatic arthritis (PA), which of the following statements is true?
   a) Findings correlate closely with corresponding symptoms.
   b) Findings correlate well with overall disease duration.
   c) Findings always precede spinal inflammatory changes.
   d) Findings are heavily integrated into PA disease classification.

The correct answer is (**b**). Many patients with PA may exhibit abnormal sacroiliac bone marrow edema on MRI. However, a large percentage of these patients are asymptomatic. MRI changes of sacroiliitis correlate well with decreased spinal mobility and longer duration of disease. Although changes of sacroiliitis frequently precede changes of spondylitis in PA patients, spondylitis may occur in the absence of sacroiliitis. Current classification criteria for PA include radiographic findings of juxta-articular new bone formation. MRI serves no current role in disease classification.

■ **Case 56**

1. Grafts used for anterior cruciate ligament (ACL) reconstruction may be harvested from which of the following structures?
   a) Sartorius
   b) Gracilis
   c) Patellar tendon
   d) All of the above
   e) None of the above

The correct answer is (**d**). The most commonly harvested tendons for ACL graft reconstruction are bone–patellar tendon–bone and hamstring autografts utilizing the semitendinosus and gracilis tendons.

2. Which of the following statements is true?
   a) Most patients with ACL graft tunnel cysts are asymptomatic.
   b) ACL tunnel cysts do not communicate with the joint.
   c) Tunnel cysts frequently cause graft failure.
   d) These cysts typically occur 10 years after the surgery.

The correct answer is (**a**). Patients with tunnel cysts are frequently asymptomatic, with findings incidentally noted on MRI. Both noncommunicating and communicating tunnel cysts have been described, with noncommunicating cysts showing no connection to the joint space. Communicating cysts demonstrate connection with the joint space, allowing synovial fluid transmission through the tunnel likely from lack of graft incorporation. Most ACL graft tunnel cysts do not cause graft failure. These cysts typically arise between 1 and 5 years after the original ACL surgery.

■ **Case 57**

1. Which of the following radiographic findings indicates arthroplasty component loosening?
   a) Stress shielding
   b) Spot welds
   c) Pedestal formation
   d) Cement mantle gas bubbles
   e) All of the above

The correct answer is (**c**). *Stress shielding* refers to the expected proximal medial femoral bone resorption occurring in the noncemented hip arthroplasty. This results from decreased stress to the proximal femoral bone stock as the distal femoral prosthesis and adjacent bone absorb loading during bone hardware ingrowth. Radiographically visible areas of sclerotic bone ingrowth may be seen abutting the noncemented femoral stem prostheses. These are referred to as *spot welds* and indicate solid fixation. Sclerotic bony changes along the femoral medullary canal just distal to the prosthetic femoral stem are related to prosthesis micromotion. These bony changes are referred to as pedestal formation. Small foci of gas bubbles within the cement mantle of the femoral component are commonly encountered. These occur during surgical implantation and are of no consequence.

2. Regarding hip hemiarthroplasty components, which of the following statement is true?
   a) The native femoral and acetabular articular surfaces are reconstructed.
   b) The native acetabular articular surface is preserved during hemiarthroplasty.
   c) Screw fixation of the acetabulum is frequently seen with hip hemiarthroplasty.
   d) Cement fixation of the acetabular component is typically seen with hemiarthroplasty.
   e) None of the above is true.

The correct answer is (**b**). Regarding hip replacement, hemiarthroplasty and total arthroplasty vary in that the femoral half of the joint is reconstructed with the former and both the femoral and acetabular joints are reconstructed with the latter. The chondral surface and underlying bone stock of the acetabulum are retained during hip hemiarthroplasty. Radiographic findings of screw fixation or cement fixation of the acetabular implant indicate total arthroplasty. These modes of acetabular fixation are utilized to secure the acetabular implant in place.

■ **Case 58**

1. Which of the following characteristics aid in the differentiation of an enchondroma from a low-grade chondrosarcoma?
    a) Internal chondroid calcifications
    b) Enhancement pattern
    c) Pain
    d) Attenuation on CT
    e) All of the above

The correct answer is (**c**). Differentiation of an enchondroma from a low-grade chondrosarcoma is crucial because surgical management is required for the latter. Most chondrosarcomas may be easily differentiated based on aggressive imaging characteristics including endosteal scalloping of greater than two thirds of the cortex along the majority of the length of the lesion, cortical destruction, periosteal reaction, pathologic fracture, and/or a soft tissue mass. A significant clinical feature associated with malignant degeneration includes the presence of pain. The presence of pain favors a diagnosis of malignancy nearly 5 times more often than enchondroma. Additionally, lesion size > 5 to 7 cm tends to favor chondrosarcoma. Chondroid calcifications, CT attenuation, and enhancement pattern are not crucial characteristics in determination of malignancy.

2. Characteristic MRI features of enchondroma include which one of the following?
    a) Spiculated morphology
    b) Hyperintense T1 and T2 signal
    c) Absence of signal voids
    d) Diffuse homogeneous enhancement
    e) None of the above

The correct answer is (**e**). Characteristic MRI findings for enchondroma include identification of a circumscribed, geographic, intramedullary region of marrow replacement demonstrating decreased signal intensity on T1 fat-sensitive sequences. Corresponding hyperintense T2 signal intensity with lobulated margins is typical. Superimposed punctate signal voids may be seen representing chondroid calcifications. Post-gadolinium imaging shows enhancement of the margins along with internal curvilinear septal enhancement.

■ **Case 59**

1. Which of the following statements regarding particle disease is true?
    a) Chronic, untreated particle disease has a moderate potential for malignant degeneration.
    b) A higher incidence of particle disease is noted in females.
    c) This process is typically confined to the effective joint space.
    d) Particle disease constitutes one of the more rare causes for revision hip arthroplasty.
    e) All of the above

The correct answer is (**c**). No malignant potential or gender predilection has been reported with particle disease. Osteolysis related to particle disease occurs anywhere along the effective joint space. The effective joint space is the entire region surrounding the joint in which particles may migrate and contact the bone. This is typically any part of the joint exposed to synovial fluid. Particle disease represents a common cause for revision hip arthroplasty.

2. Regarding CT imaging of particle disease, which of the following findings is expected?
    a) Poorly defined lucencies with fluid attenuation abutting the arthroplasty components
    b) Fluid-filled cysts with sclerotic borders abutting the prosthesis
    c) Circumscribed lobulated lucencies continuous with the prosthesis with soft tissue attenuation
    d) Fluid-filled periprosthetic cysts containing shards of calcific debris

The correct answer is (**c**). CT findings of particle disease include circumscribed, periprosthetic, osteolytic locules composed of soft tissue density. The internal soft tissue density is secondary to granulomatous change related to the immune response incited by the shed polyethylene particles. These findings communicate with the joint capsule.

■ **Case 60**

1. Which of the following is felt to represent the underlying abnormality associated with fibrodysplasia ossificans progressiva (FOP)?
    a) Subclinical bleeding disorder
    b) Bone morphogenetic protein dysfunction
    c) Autoimmune process
    d) Immunoglobulin deficiency
    e) None of the above

The correct answer is (**b**). The bone morphogenetic protein is hypothesized to play a role in this disorder. Although no distinct mutation has been identified, research suggests upregulation and/or dysfunction in this protein allowing for overexpression and overproduction of bone formation.

2. Which of the following statements regarding bone formation in FOP is true?
   a) The mechanism is similar to myositis ossificans.
   b) A zonal pattern of heterotopic ossification is typical.
   c) Enchondral ossification represents the primary mode of bone formation.
   d) All of the above are true.
   e) None of the above are true.

The correct answer is (**c**). The development of bone formation in this disorder follows an orderly progression. An inflammatory soft tissue intramuscular reaction represents the initial change. Highly vascular stromal tissue then develops which gives rise to a hyaline cartilage intermediate with subsequent ossification, likened to enchondral ossification. The typical zonal pattern of ossification is not seen with this disease process.

■ Case 61

1. Giant cell tumor (GCT) of the tendon sheath shares similar MRI characteristics with which of the following?
   a) Pigmented villonodular synovitis
   b) Clear cell sarcoma
   c) Nodular fasciitis
   d) Intramuscular myxoma
   e) None of the above

The correct answer is (**a**). Pigmented villonodular synovitis is a neoplasm exhibiting similar histologic features to GCT of the tendon sheath. Both lesions histologically display chronic inflammatory cells that contain hemosiderin, accounting for the low T1/T2 signal and blooming artifact on MRI.

2. Which of the following statements regarding GCT of the tendon sheath is true?
   a) These lesions are frequently multifocal.
   b) Radiographic findings of calcification are fairly typical.
   c) These lesions are frequently predated by trauma.
   d) These are relatively vascular masses exhibiting post-gadolinium enhancement on MRI and increased color flow on ultrasound.
   e) None of the above

The correct answer is (**d**). Although giant cell tumor of the tendon sheath has been reported to be multifocal, most lesions are solitary. These lesions are fairly vascular and exhibit avid enhancement following gadolinium administration on MRI. Color Doppler flow typically demonstrates increased vascularity on ultrasound imaging. Calcifications are typically not detected on radiographs. No association with trauma has been reported.

■ Case 62

1. Features typical of focal intra-articular pigmented villonodular synovitis (PVNS) include which one of the following?
   a) Single area of synovial thickening at arthrography
   b) Hemorrhagic arthrocentesis
   c) Focal hypermetabolic activity on positron emission tomography (PET)/CT scanning
   d) All of the above
   e) None of the above

The correct answer is (**d**). Whereas arthrography of the diffuse variant of PVNS reveals extensive synovial thickening with nodular projections, localized PVNS may show a single nodular area of synovial thickening. The typical fluid aspirated from the knee of the patient with focal PVNS is bloody. Focal PVNS may reveal hypermetabolic activity with fluorine-18 fluorodeoxyglucose PET/CT imaging.

2. Which of the following is a distinguishing feature between focal and diffuse PVNS?
   a) Focal PVNS more frequently shows a frondlike appearance of the synovium.
   b) A large-sized effusion is more typical of focal PVNS.
   c) Focal PVNS is typically sessile in relation to the synovium.
   d) Hemosiderin deposition is less abundant with focal PVNS.
   e) Recurrence rate following resection of these two entities is equal.

The correct answer is (**d**). Histologically, generalized and focal PVNS are similar. The MR features and clinical course of the diffuse versus focal form are different. Generalized PVNS more frequently displays a frondlike synovial pattern with more abundant hemosiderin deposition. Focal PVNS is typically a pedunculated synovial lesion. A large effusion is typical for generalized PVNS, whereas it is more atypical for focal PVNS. Total synovectomy is required treatment for the generalized form of PVNS, with varying rates of significant recurrence. Local resection of focal PVNS is typically curative, with rare recurrence.

■ Case 63

1. Regarding the anatomy and function of the posterior interosseous nerve, which statement is correct?
   a) This is a sensory branch of the radial nerve.
   b) This is a sensory branch of the musculocutaneous nerve.
   c) This is a posterior motor branch of the radial nerve.
   d) This is a motor branch of the median nerve.

The correct answer is (**c**). The radial nerve arises from the posterior cord of the brachial plexus and follows the brachial artery proximally. The nerve bifurcates at the level of the lateral epicondyle adjacent to the elbow, forming a deep motor branch. This segment of the nerve pierces the supinator muscle anteriorly and exits posteriorly as the posterior interosseous nerve.

2. The normal MR appearance of peripheral nerves includes which of the following?
    a) Hypointense T1 and intermediate to mildly hyperintense T2 signal with uniform size
    b) Fusiform morphology
    c) Hyperintense T1 and T2 signal
    d) Peripheral enhancement following gadolinium administration
    e) None of the above

The correct answer is (**a**). The normal MRI appearance of peripheral nerves on fat-sensitive axial T1 imaging includes a smooth round/ovoid structure with signal isointense to muscle. Normal T2 signal characteristics include isointensity to mild hyperintensity relative to normal muscle. Lack of enhancement should be observed following contrast administration. Axial imaging planes are ideal for evaluating neural anatomy in the extremities given the nerve size and orientation. There should be uniformity in the size of the nerve along its longitudinal course. Any deviation from these signal characteristics or structural features should imply nerve pathology.

■ Case 64

1. All of the following are associated with motion artifact, except...
    a) Swallowing
    b) Breathing
    c) Peristalsis
    d) Paresthesias
    e) None of the above

The correct answer is (**d**). Motion artifact may extend across the entire field of view, occurring as a result of movement during image acquisition. These artifacts are seen with pulsation from arterial structures, respiration, peristalsis, swallowing, or extrinsic patient motion. Paresthesias do not result in detectable motion artifact.

2. Which of the following anatomic structures are prone to distortion as a result of pulsation artifact?
    a) The articular cartilage of the hip and patellofemoral joints
    b) The carpal tunnel
    c) The thumb metacarpophalangeal joint collateral ligaments
    d) The peroneal tendons
    e) None of the above

The correct answer is (**a**). Phasing encoding pulsation artifact on axial images may occur at the level of the patellofemoral and femoral acetabular joints secondary to potential in-plane imaging artifact from the popliteal and femoral arteries, respectively. Ghosting artifact created from pulsation of the popliteal and femoral arteries may be superimposed over the hyaline cartilage of these articulations, limiting accurate evaluation.

■ Case 65

1. Which of the following syndromes is associated with fibrous dysplasia?
    a) McCune–Albright syndrome
    b) Maffucci syndrome
    c) Jaffe–Campanacci syndrome
    d) Osler–Weber–Rendu syndrome
    e) All of the above

The correct answer is (**a**). McCune–Albright syndrome consists of precocious puberty, polyostotic fibrous dysplasia, with café au lait spots resembling the coast of Maine. This disease process is primarily seen in females and may be associated with endocrinopathies. An additional condition associated with fibrous dysplasia is Mazabraud syndrome, which is represented by a combination of fibrous dysplasia and soft tissue myxomas.

2. Which of the following statements regarding the malignant potential of fibrous dysplasia is true?
    a) No malignant potential exists.
    b) Malignancy occurs in < 1% of cases.
    c) Twenty percent of polyostotic fibrous dysplasia converts to malignancy.
    d) None of the above statements is true.

The correct answer is (**b**). Malignant degeneration of fibrous dysplasia is rare, occurring in ~1% of all cases. These patients may present with pain and swelling with radiographs demonstrating cortical destruction with soft tissue masses. Malignant transformation has been described in both polyostotic and monostotic variants of fibrous dysplasia. The most common malignancies include osteosarcoma and fibrosarcoma.

■ Case 66

1. All of the following are major contributors to patellar instability, except...
    a) Trochlea dysplasia
    b) Lateral distance between the tibial tubercle and trochlea groove
    c) Femoral cam deformity
    d) Patella alta
    e) None of the above

The correct answer is (**c**). Primary components predisposing to patellar instability include a shallow or dysplastic trochlea, a lateralized tibial tubercle of > 2 cm relative to the trochlear groove, and a high-riding patella, or patella alta. The shallow trochlear notch does not allow for optimal engagement and optimal tracking of the patella. A lateralized tibial tuberosity results in excessive lateral traction upon the patella from the patellar tendon. A high-riding patella requires a greater degree of flexion to engage the patella within the trochlear notch. Femoral cam deformity is not implicated with patellar instability.

2. Injury to the medial patellofemoral retinaculum following lateral patellofemoral dislocation occurs most commonly at which location?
   a) The patellar insertional fibers
   b) The femoral insertional fibers
   c) The mid-substance fibers
   d) Multifocal ligamentous injury is most common
   e) None of the above

The correct answer is (**a**). The most important stabilizers of the patellofemoral joint are the medial patellofemoral retinaculum and medial patellofemoral ligament. Fifty to 90% of patients with prior lateral patellofemoral dislocation demonstrate injury to these structures at the patellar insertional fibers. Characterization of the site of injury is crucial because patients with femoral avulsion injuries have an increased risk of chronic instability.

■ Case 67

1. Distinguishing features between synovial thickening and a joint effusion on MR imaging include which of the following?
   a) Joint effusion is heterogeneously bright on T2-weighted sequences.
   b) Synovial thickening demonstrates intermediate soft tissue T2 signal.
   c) Synovial thickening demonstrates rim enhancement.
   d) A joint effusion will typically demonstrate solid enhancement.
   e) None of the above

The correct answer is (**b**). Differentiating a joint effusion from synovial thickening may be challenging on MRI, particularly in smaller volume joints. Characteristic findings of a joint effusion include hypointense T1 and uniform, homogeneous, hyperintense T2 signal. Contrast administration demonstrates synovial rim enhancement surrounding the joint effusion. However, a marked delay in imaging after contrast administration may allow diffusion of gadolinium from the synovium into the joint space causing diffusely increased T1 signal within the entire effusion. Synovial tissue lines the joint capsule and is typically not detectable on MRI in the absence of synovial thickening.

However, extensive neovascularization of the tissue, as seen with rheumatoid arthritis (RA), results in thickening of the synovium. Synovial thickening on MRI manifests as intermediate T2 signal extending into the joint capsule. This thickened tissue displays avid, solid enhancement following gadolinium administration.

2. Features differentiating tuberculous arthritis from RA in the knee joint include which of the following?
   a) Osteopenia and synovial thickening are not seen with tuberculous arthritis.
   b) Aggressive joint space loss and large erosions are more typical of rheumatoid arthropathy.
   c) Rice bodies are characteristic of rheumatoid arthropathy.
   d) All of the above
   e) None of the above

The correct answer is (**e**). Both tuberculous arthropathy and RA have a relatively chronic course composed of periarticular soft tissue swelling, periarticular osteopenia, bone erosions, joint effusions, and synovial thickening with gradual joint space loss. Both conditions are also reported to contain intracapsular rice bodies. These bodies represent fibrous subcentimeter nodules that exhibit low signal on MRI. The synovial thickening in rheumatoid arthropathy tends to be thicker, lobulated, and uneven, whereas the synovial thickening in tuberculous arthropathy is more uniform and less bulky. Tuberculous arthropathy exhibits more irregular and large bony erosions.

■ Case 68

1. Which of the following may predispose to patella tendinopathy?
   a) Rheumatoid arthritis
   b) Lupus
   c) Seronegative spondyloarthropathies
   d) Fluoroquinolones
   e) All of the above

The correct answer is (**e**). In addition to mechanical causes of patellar tendinopathy, systemic, inflammatory, and metabolic causes may serve as causes of tendinopathy. Specifically, rheumatoid arthritis, seronegative spondyloarthropathies, steroid use, metabolic bone disease (renal osteodystrophy), lupus, and fluoroquinolone usage have been linked to tendinopathy at various sites in the human body.

2. Which of the following regarding patellar tendon anatomy is false?
   a) Contains a tendon sheath
   b) Bordered distally by a bursa
   c) A component of the extensor mechanism
   d) Originates from the patellar cortex and inserts upon the tibial tuberosity
   e) None of the above

The correct answer is (**a**). The patellar tendon does not contain a tendon sheath. The distal patellar tendon is bordered by the deep infrapatellar bursa posteriorly. The patellar tendon represents a component of the extensor mechanism, combined with the quadriceps tendon, and is actively involved with flexion and extension of the knee along with patellofemoral tracking. This tendon arises from the anterior inferior margin of the patellar cortex inserting distally at the tibial tuberosity.

■ Case 69

1. Which of the following MR sequences may provide assistance with detecting a pathologic fracture?
   a) Elastography
   b) Diffusion-weighted imaging
   c) Gradient echo imaging
   d) Tractography
   e) None of the above

The correct answer is (**b**). Diffusion-weighted MR imaging utilizes the physics principal of Brownian motion. This states that extracellular water molecules may freely diffuse, as is the usual scenario in the normal bone marrow environment. Conversely, restricted diffusion is seen with intracellular water molecules, which are in abundance with higher cellularity bone marrow malignancies. As a result, the marrow site at a pathologic fracture may display diminished diffusion and increased MR signal, as opposed to the typical nonpathologic fracture. However, sensitivity and specificity of these diffusion-weighted MRI signal changes are variable. These findings should be interpreted in conjunction with conventional MR imaging sequences for the appropriate diagnosis of a pathologic intramedullary process.

2. The expected normal bone marrow MR signal changes in the adult appendicular skeleton include which of the following?
   a) Increased T1 and T2 signal
   b) Increased T1 and decreased T2 signal
   c) Decreased T1 and decreased T2 signal
   d) Intermediate T1 and increased T2 signal
   e) None of the above

The correct answer is (**b**). In the healthy adult skeleton, hematopoiesis is primarily confined to the calvarium, vertebra, metaphysis of long bones, and the pelvis. These sites remain active in red cell production throughout adult life. The vast majority of the healthy adult appendicular skeleton is filled with fat. As a result, the marrow exhibits increased T1 and decreased T2 signal intensity on MRI imaging. These MRI signal changes may be altered by any process requiring increased red blood cell production, most commonly anemia. Other potential causes for MR signal alteration within the bone marrow include metastases or primary bone marrow malignancies such as myeloma and leukemia.

■ Case 70

1. Which of the following is the best discriminating factor between telangiectatic osteosarcoma and aneurysmal bone cyst?
   a) Fluid–fluid levels with medullary expansion
   b) Infiltrative growth pattern, periosteal reaction, and osteolysis
   c) Metaphyseal location and pathologic fracture
   d) Lytic long bone lesion with pain upon presentation

The correct answer is (**b**). Osteolysis, an infiltrative soft tissue mass, and periosteal reaction are the best discriminating features between telangiectatic osteosarcoma and aneurysmal bone cyst. Both lesions exhibit fluid–fluid levels related to internal hemorrhage. Aneurysmal bone cysts may present with pathologic fractures causing pain upon presentation. Both aneurysmal bone cyst and telangiectatic osteosarcoma may present as a lytic long bone metaphyseal lesion.

2. Which of the following statements regarding telangiectatic osteosarcoma is false?
   a) This subtype of osteosarcoma is less aggressive than parosteal osteosarcoma.
   b) Biopsy of the soft tissue component provides the highest chance for an accurate diagnosis.
   c) This variant of osteosarcoma typically presents in the 2nd and 3rd decades of life.
   d) This tumor has an equivalent or more favorable survival rate when compared with conventional osteosarcoma.

The correct answer is (**a**). Multiple subtypes of osteosarcoma exist. Conventional parosteal osteosarcoma is a surface osteosarcoma. This subtype has a more favorable prognosis when compared with other osteosarcoma variants, with expected survival rates of ~90% following surgical resection only. Tissue sampling from the solid soft tissue mass component of telangiectatic osteosarcoma provides the highest diagnostic yield. Accurate diagnosis and differentiation from conventional osteosarcoma is important for treatment and prognosis. Emerging research is demonstrating improved survival for patients with telangiectatic osteosarcoma in comparison to patients with conventional osteosarcoma. The typical patient presenting with telangiectatic osteosarcoma is in the 2nd or 3rd decade of life.

■ Case 71

1. Secondary findings of an anterior cruciate ligament (ACL) tear include which of the following?
   a) "Uncoverage" of the posterior horn of the lateral meniscus
   b) Vertical orientation of the fibular collateral ligament
   c) Vertical tear along the red zone of the posterior horn medial meniscus adjacent to the root insertion
   d) Posterior horn lateral meniscal tear along the plane of the meniscofemoral ligament
   e) All of the above

The correct answer is (**e**). Rupture of the ACL results in anterior positioning of the tibia relative to the femur. This alignment shift results in uncoverage of the posterior horn lateral meniscus and vertical orientation of the fibular collateral ligament. This new orientation of the fibular collateral ligament allows for near complete visualization of this structure on a single coronal MR image. Additionally, posterior horn tearing of the medial and lateral menisci in a vertical oblique fashion is seen. This may occur at the level of the posterior horn lateral meniscus along the plane of the meniscofemoral ligament and along the peripheral vascular red zone of the posterior horn medial meniscus. Other secondary features of ACL tears include buckling of the posterior cruciate ligament and tears of the posterior capsule, arcuate ligament, and medial collateral ligament.

2. Which of the following represents the anatomic composition of the ACL?
   a) Anteromedial and posterolateral ligamentous bundles
   b) A single ligamentous bundle
   c) Anterolateral and posteromedial ligamentous bundles
   d) A solitary thick tendinous bundle
   e) All of the above

The correct answer is (**a**). The ACL is composed of dense ligamentous tissue containing anteromedial and posterolateral bundles. Of these two bundles, the anteromedial component is most important for stability and is under tension upon flexion. The posterolateral component falls under tension upon extension. The anteromedial bundle is most commonly implicated with partial ACL tears or sprains.

■ Case 72

1. Expected MRI findings in patients with ankylosing spondylitis (AS) with cervical spine injury include which of the following?
   a) Longitudinal ligamentous disruption
   b) Multilevel vertebral body compression fractures
   c) Cord contusion
   d) Both a and c
   e) Both b and c

The correct answer is (**d**). MRI is ideally suited for evaluation of cervical spine soft tissue injuries in patients with AS. These injuries typically involve all three columns and may involve fractures of the vertebral bodies, facets, and spinous processes. In addition, disruption of the anterior and posterior longitudinal ligaments may be demonstrated with a fracture extending through the ossified disk space. Abnormal spinal cord signal secondary to contusion or cord transection may be seen. Multilevel vertebral body compression fractures are atypical in these patients, given the relatively fixated and rigid spine.

2. Other typical findings in patients with AS include which of the following?
   a) Bridging symmetric syndesmophyte formation in the thoracic and lumbar spine
   b) Unilateral sacroiliac joint fusion
   c) Subluxation of the metacarpophalangeal joints
   d) Multifocal avascular necrosis
   e) None of the above

The correct answer is (**a**). AS is a chronic inflammatory condition primarily affecting the axial skeletal entheses and cartilaginous/synovial based joints. Erosions followed by bone formation and fusion at these various sites in the skeleton may occur. Typical features of this disease include symmetric bilateral sacroiliitis with eventual fusion along with diffuse symmetric bridging syndesmophyte formation involving the entire spine. Subluxations involving the joints of the hands and avascular necrosis are not typical features of this disease.

■ Case 73

1. All of the following conditions are expected to show increased intramuscular fluid signal intensity on MR imaging, except...
   a) Acute denervation
   b) Acute polymyositis
   c) Chronic denervation
   d) Muscle contusion

The correct answer is (**c**). Acute muscle denervation results in geographic T2 signal increase within the affected denervated muscle group. This is thought to reflect a shift of water from the intracellular to the extracellular space.

Chronic muscle denervation results in fatty infiltration of musculature and does not display intramuscular T2 signal increase. Polymyositis is an immune-driven inflammatory process affecting striated skeletal muscle. Typical acute MRI findings include bilateral symmetric T2 signal increase in the pelvic and thigh musculature. Chronic polymyositis manifests with fatty infiltration of the musculature. Muscle contusions result from a direct blow to the musculature, with MR imaging demonstrating intramuscular T2 signal increase secondary to interstitial hemorrhaging.

2. Which of the following anatomic regions are particularly prone to compartment syndrome and muscle infarction?
    a) Forearm and leg
    b) Thigh and forefoot
    c) Shoulder girdle musculature
    d) Gluteal musculature
    e) None of the above

The correct answer is (**a**). Although compartment syndrome and muscle infarcts have been reported in the foot, thigh, and gluteal regions, the most common sites in the human skeleton are the leg and forearm. These sites contain tight and unyielding fascial compartments, which are particularly prone to muscle infarction. The anterior compartment of the leg serves as the most common location for acute compartment syndrome and contains the extensor musculature of the foot.

■ Case 74

1. Which of the following muscles are expected to be injured with scapulothoracic dissociation (STD)?
    a) Deltoid
    b) Pectoralis
    c) Trapezius
    d) Latissimus dorsi
    e) All of the above

The correct answer is (**e**). Articulations of the shoulder include the glenohumeral joint, the acromioclavicular joint, and the scapulothoracic articulation. The shoulder girdle musculature serves as a dynamic stabilizer of these articulations. STD represents a complete separation of the scapula from the thorax, with disruption of the associated dynamic stabilizers. Associated injuries to the shoulder girdle musculature are frequent and involve the deltoid, pectoralis minor, rhomboid, levator scapula, trapezius, and latissimus dorsi.

2. Brachial plexus injury implicates which of the following nerves?
    a) C3–C8
    b) C4–C7
    c) C8–T2
    d) C5–T1
    e) None of the above

The correct answer is (**d**). The brachial plexus is composed of nerves originating from the lower cervical and upper thoracic nerve roots. This plexus is responsible for innervating musculature and skin of the shoulder and arm. C5–T1 make up the brachial plexus and are divided into trunks, divisions, cords, branches, and nerves. Injury to these structures is not uncommon with STD.

■ Case 75

1. Which of the following represents the distinguishing feature between reactive arthritis and psoriatic arthritis (PA)?
    a) PA has an association with genitourinary infections.
    b) PA has a predilection for both the upper and lower extremities, whereas reactive arthritis more commonly affects the lower extremities.
    c) Reactive arthritis typically causes profound osteopenia.
    d) Sacroiliitis is not a feature of PA.
    e) None of the above

The correct answer is (**b**). Contrary to PA, reactive arthritis is preceded by an enteric or urogenital infectious process. Both entities cause osseous erosive and proliferative changes in the upper and lower extremities; however, osseous changes in reactive arthritis are more frequently seen in the lower extremities. Significant osteopenia is not a consistent feature of either reactive arthritis or PA. PA and reactive arthritis both affect the axial skeleton, causing asymmetric sacroiliitis with subchondral bone plate erosions and irregularity.

2. MRI features of PA arthritis in the hand typically include which of the following?
    a) Tenosynovitis
    b) Bone marrow edema
    c) Rice bodies
    d) All of the above
    e) Both a and b

The correct answer is (**e**). Typical MRI features of the hand in patients with PA include enthesitis manifesting as multifocal bone marrow edema and enhancement at capsular, ligamentous, and tendinous bony insertions. Tenosynovitis with subcutaneous edema and enhancement are also seen during active inflammation with PA. Rice bodies are not a feature of PA in the hands.

Case 76

1. Which of the following statements is true?
   a) Chromium cobalt prostheses are more commonly associated with metallosis.
   b) Metal debris from arthroplasty components is biologically inert.
   c) Treatment for early metallosis is not required.
   d) An intense inflammatory response may be seen with polyethylene and metallic debris.
   e) All of the above are true.

The correct answer is (**d**). Titanium components appear to be more commonly associated with metallosis than other metallic arthroplasty components. Metallic debris from arthroplasty components is not biologically inert. This debris incites a synovial inflammatory response related to macrophage activation and may cause implant loosening with osteolysis. This inflammation is intensified with the concomitant release of polyethylene particles. Early treatment for metallosis is recommended to prevent progressive osteolysis and soft tissue damage. Treatment includes resection of the affected soft tissues/synovium with hardware revision.

2. Regarding imaging of metallosis, which of the following statements is true?
   a) Metallosis is always visible on radiographs.
   b) MR imaging of bony changes adjacent to arthroplasty components is optimized by increasing receiver bandwidth.
   c) Gradient echo MR imaging may assist with confirming the diagnosis.
   d) Dual-energy CT scanning offers minimal advantage in the evaluation of metallosis.
   e) None of the above is true.

The correct answer is (**c**). Metallosis is frequently, but not always, visible on radiography. Modifications of MR imaging to optimize evaluation of bony changes adjacent to arthroplasty components include decreasing voxel size, utilization of fast spin-echo imaging, and decreasing the receiver bandwidth. Gradient echo MR imaging may degrade image quality in the presence of hardware secondary to extensive blooming artifact. However, utilization of this sequence in the setting of metallosis allows detection of metal debris within the synovium and adjacent soft tissues. Dual-energy CT scanning allows optimal detection of metallosis-induced osteolysis at the bone–hardware interface by minimizing beam hardening/streak artifact.

Case 77

1. All of the following statements regarding olecranon bursitis are true, except…
   a) Also referred to as student's elbow or miner's elbow
   b) May coexist with amorphous MRI signal voids
   c) MRI may show fluid demonstrating increased T1 and increased T2 signal
   d) May lead to rupture of the triceps tendon
   e) All of the above are true

The correct answer is (**e**). Olecranon bursitis is synonymous with student's elbow or miner's elbow. Olecranon bursitis may coexist with gout, in which case crystalline deposits may be identified exhibiting diminished T1 and T2 signal on MR imaging. Hemorrhagic bursitis may manifest with increased T1 and increased T2 signal secondary to extracellular methemoglobin. Chronic olecranon bursal inflammation may lead to weakening of the triceps tendon with eventual rupture. Following the administration of contrast, the olecranon bursa typically exhibits rim enhancement secondary to its synovial lining.

2. Other bursae commonly seen at the level of the elbow include which of the following?
   a) Medial collateral ligament bursa
   b) Epicondylar bursa
   c) Bicipital radial bursa
   d) Coronoid bursa
   e) None of the above

The correct answer is (**c**). The bicipital radial bursa lies at the level of the distal biceps tendon adjacent to the radial tuberosity insertion. This bursa may become inflamed as a result of distal biceps tendinopathy.

Case 78

1. Potential causes of humeral head cystic bony changes include all the following except…
   a) Hydroxyapatite deposition
   b) Gout
   c) Adhesive capsulitis
   d) Osteoarthrosis
   e) Posterior superior shoulder impingement

The correct answer is (**c**). Calcium hydroxyapatite deposition at the level of the shoulder joint may exist in an intraosseous phase. During this phase, calcific deposits migrate and erode into the humeral head, manifesting radiographically with subcortical cystic changes with or without detectable calcific deposits. Periarticular and para-articular gouty deposits may be deposited within the humeral head, manifesting radiographically as intraosseous cysts with or without detectable crystals. Adhesive capsulitis is an idiopathic self-limiting inflammatory condition of the anterior–inferior joint capsule not typically known for causing cystic changes within the humeral head. Osteoarthritis represents a degenerative overuse condition with classic radiographic features of joint space narrowing, subchondral sclerosis, and marginal osteophyte formation, with or without subcortical cystic changes. Posterior and superior shoulder impingement represents an internal impingement disorder at the glenohumeral joint, typically seen in the throwing shoulder. Characteristic findings include posterior supraspinatus and anterior infraspinatus tendon undersurface tearing with underlying greater tuberosity cystic changes.

2. An enthesis represents which of the following?
    a) The interface at the bony insertion of ligaments and tendons
    b) The transition of muscle to tendon
    c) The segment of tendon within the central skeletal muscle belly
    d) A synovial-lined sac present between tendon and underlying bone
    e) None of the above

The correct answer is (**a**). An enthesis represents the site of tendon or ligament attachment to bone. This site may be affected by inflammatory conditions, trauma, or degeneration, among other etiologies. Seronegative spondyloarthropathies serve as a frequent cause of inflammation at these sites, termed enthesitis. Radiographic manifestations of enthesitis include erosions as well as sclerosis with subsequent bone formation characteristically seen along the spine, the sacroiliac joints, the greater trochanters of the femora, and the humeral head greater tuberosities.

■ Case 79

1. "Wolff's law" refers to which of the following?
    a) Adaptive responses of bone
    b) Compensatory muscle hypertrophy
    c) Metabolic bone disease
    d) Blood pressure and resistance increase with diameter decrease
    e) None of the above

The correct answer is (**a**). Wolff's law is fundamental in understanding fatigue and insufficiency fractures. Simply stated, cortical and trabeculated bone respond to their mechanical environment. As external force is applied to bone, cortical trabecular remodeling and hypertrophy ensue. These changes are detectable on radiography as cortical thickening and medullary sclerosis. Alternatively, as cortical and trabeculated bone are off-loaded or unchallenged by external forces for an extended period of time, bony atrophy occurs. This results in osteopenia on radiography.

2. Which of the following is a common site for insufficiency fractures?
    a) Scapula
    b) Femur
    c) Sacrum
    d) Tibia
    e) All of the above

The correct answer is (**e**). The scapula, femur, sacrum, and tibia all represent common sites prone to insufficiency fractures. These patients typically have postmenopausal osteoporosis or chronic renal disease associated with metabolic bone disease. The sacrum typically demonstrates vertically oriented fractures, whereas transverse fractures are seen through the proximal medial tibial metaphysis, the lateral margin of the scapular neck, and the femoral neck. Femoral head and femoral condylar insufficiency fractures typically parallel the adjacent articular surfaces.

■ Case 80

1. Regarding MRI findings of rheumatoid arthritis (RA), which of the following statements is true?
    a) Erosions are not detectable on MRI.
    b) Tenosynovitis is unusual.
    c) Marrow edema may serve as a surrogate marker for inflammation.
    d) All of the above are true.
    e) None of the above is true.

The correct answer is (**c**). MRI is emerging as an important imaging modality in the evaluation of RA. Periarticular bony erosions are detectable with this modality. Erosive changes are best displayed on T1-weighted imaging and should be located in a periarticular distribution and visualized in two separate imaging planes. Fluid and synovial thickening frequently distend the tendon sheaths in the early stages of RA. MR imaging demonstrates T2 signal increase with soft tissue fullness within the affected tendon sheaths. Subchondral bone marrow edema is considered to be a very early marker of inflammation and is closely related to the degree of synovitis.

2. Current criteria for classifying RA include which of the following imaging modalities?
    a) Radiographs
    b) Ultrasound
    c) MRI
    d) All of the above

The correct answer is (**a**). Classification criteria for RA set forth by the American College of Rheumatology include radiographic changes of periarticular erosions and osteopenia. These criteria are combined with multiple clinical and serologic findings. Although MRI and ultrasound do not have established roles in the routine evaluation of patients with polyarthritis, these imaging modalities are more sensitive than radiography at detecting changes from synovitis and may be helpful in quantifying synovial inflammation.

■ Case 81

1. The two most commonly associated variants related to patellofemoral maltracking and fat pad impingement include which of the following?
    a) Genu varus and trochlear hypoplasia
    b) Lateral distance between the tibial tubercle–trochlea groove and patella alta
    c) Genu valgus and patella alta
    d) Patella baja and trochlear hypoplasia
    e) None of the above

The correct answer is (**b**). Patellofemoral maltracking is believed to be strongly related to a high-riding patella and an increased tibial tuberosity–trochlear groove distance. These two variants are also highly associated with lateral patellofemoral subluxation. A lateralized tibial tuberosity results in excessive lateral traction upon the patella from the patellar tendon. A lateralized tibial tubercle of > 2 cm relative to the trochlear groove is considered pathologic. A high-riding patella requires a greater degree of flexion to engage the patella within the trochlear notch, allowing for dynamic instability and maltracking.

2. Which the following structures serve as an anatomic border of Hoffa's fat?
    a) The patellofemoral retinacula
    b) The anterior cruciate ligament
    c) The deep infrapatellar bursa
    d) The transverse meniscal ligament
    e) All of the above

The correct answer is (**c**). Hoffa's fat, or the deep infrapatellar fat, is bordered by the inferior pole of the patella superiorly, the anterior proximal tibia and deep infrapatellar bursa inferiorly, the synovial lining of the joint cavity posteriorly, and the joint capsule and patellar tendon anteriorly.

■ Case 82

1. Imaging features allowing distinction of avascular necrosis from transient migratory bone marrow edema include which of the following?
    a) Central photopenia within the femoral head may be seen with avascular necrosis.
    b) The "double line" sign is a unique finding for avascular necrosis.
    c) Bone marrow signal changes are more homogeneous with transient bone marrow edema.
    d) Bone marrow signal alterations are more diffuse in distribution within the femoral head and neck with transient marrow edema.
    e) All of the above

The correct answer is (**e**). Radionuclide bone scan is typically cold in the early stages of avascular necrosis related to the bone marrow infarct. This differs from transient bone marrow edema which exhibits increased radionuclide uptake in the femoral head early on in the disease process. MRI changes of femoral head avascular necrosis include the "double line" sign, which is not a feature of transient marrow edema. This sign is represented by femoral head T2 signal characteristics of a peripheral low-signal zone related to reactive bone formation surrounding an internal high-signal zone related to the cellular vascular reparative process. A circumscribed, subchondral, bandlike low T1 signal intensity line has also been described in the femoral head with avascular necrosis. Transient bone marrow edema changes on MRI include diffuse and homogeneous diminished T1 and increased T2 signal distributed throughout the femoral head and neck, terminating at the level of joint capsular insertion.

2. In addition to transient bone marrow edema of the hip, additional causes of osteopenia at the level of the hip joint include which of the following?
    a) Reflex sympathetic dystrophy
    b) Rheumatoid arthritis
    c) Calcium pyrophosphate dihydrate disease (CPPD) arthropathy
    d) All of the above
    e) Both a and b

The correct answer is (**e**). Reflex sympathetic dystrophy represents a pain syndrome characterized by localized dull and burning pain with superimposed sensorimotor alterations. Radiographic findings include severe patchy and periarticular osteopenia involving the affected area, with soft tissue swelling. Rheumatoid arthritis represents a chronic, symmetric, and erosive inflammatory arthropathy with characteristic hip radiographic findings of periarticular osteopenia and/or osteoporosis superimposed upon uniform femoral acetabular joint space loss. CPPD arthropathy is a crystalline-driven arthritis that may affect the hip joint. However, osteopenia is not a typical feature of this arthropathy.

■ Case 83

1. Distinguishing features between calcium pyrophosphate crystal deposition (CPPD) arthropathy and osteoarthrosis of the knee joint include which of the following?
    a) Absence of medial femoral tibial compartment involvement with CPPD arthropathy
    b) Extensive subcortical cyst formation with osteoarthrosis
    c) Absence of patellofemoral involvement with osteoarthrosis
    d) Periarticular and intra-articular calcific deposits with CPPD arthropathy
    e) None of the above

The correct answer is (**d**). Features differentiating CPPD arthropathy from osteoarthritis of the knee include the joint compartment distribution. CPPD arthropathy may commonly involve the medial femoral tibial compartment. However, isolated patellofemoral arthropathy of the knee joint should suggest this disease process. This is particularly true in older patients, even in the absence of crystalline deposits. Subcortical cyst formation may be seen with severe osteoarthritis. However, extensive subchondral cyst formation is more typical with CPPD arthropathy and is related to the superimposed calcium deposits. Medial knee compartment joint space loss with sclerosis and osteophyte formation are the signature findings with osteoarthrosis because this is the major weight-bearing compartment of the knee. However, milder arthritic involvement of the patellofemoral compartment is also a feature of osteoarthrosis. Periarticular and intra-articular calcific deposits are extremely common with CPPD arthropathy. Sites of crystalline deposits include the menisci, hyaline cartilage, suprapatellar bursa, posterior capsule, gastrocnemius tendons, and quadriceps tendon. Of note, the posterior hyaline cartilage of the knee joint is more commonly affected with chondrocalcinosis.

2. Expected MRI findings of CPPD in hyaline cartilage include which of the following?
    a) Linear and punctate hyperintense T1/T2 signal
    b) Globular hyperintense T1/T2 signal
    c) Linear and punctate hypointense T1/T2 signal
    d) No detectable abnormality on MR imaging
    e) All of the above

The correct answer is (**c**). Articular hyaline cartilage deposits of CPPD may be detectable on MR imaging. These deposits may be present along the surface or middle layer of the hyaline cartilage, appearing as thin, linear, or punctate regions of hypointense T1 and T2 signal. These deposits parallel the subchondral bone plate. A surrounding halo of signal increase may be seen around these deposits secondary to susceptibility artifact. Blooming artifact from cartilage CPPD deposits may be elicited by deploying gradient echo MR imaging.

■ Case 84

1. Regarding the pathophysiology of Freiberg's infraction, which of the following statements is true?
    a) Second metatarsal head involvement occurs as a result of disproportionate load-bearing through this ray.
    b) Abnormal alignment of the hallux metatarsal increases the risk for this disease process.
    c) Flatfoot deformity predisposes to this condition.
    d) Plantar fascial abnormalities typically coexist and may be a root cause of this disorder.
    e) Both a and d

The correct answer is (**a**). The second and third metatarsals are most frequently implicated with Freiberg's infraction. This likely relates to a combination of factors. These metatarsals represent the longest of the five metatarsals. As a result, absorption of the majority of forefoot force upon ambulation occurs at these sites, predisposing these metatarsal heads to excess trauma. Additionally, the second and third metatarsals are less mobile than the remaining metatarsals, allowing less ability to displace force upon ambulation.

2. Which of the following statements regarding metatarsal head blood supply is true?
    a) No direct blood supply exists to the metatarsal epiphyses.
    b) Dual arterial blood supply to the metatarsal epiphyses exists.
    c) Single arterial blood supply to the metatarsal epiphyses exists.
    d) Watershed arterial supply to the second and third metatarsal heads exists.
    e) None of the above is true.

The correct answer is (**b**). A rich blood supply exists to the metatarsal epiphyses. This occurs through anastomotic dorsal and plantar metatarsal arterial branches from the dorsalis pedis and posterior tibial arteries, respectively. Traumatic end-artery disruption of these branches may occur in the developing skeleton, predisposing patients to Freiberg's infraction.

■ Case 85

1. Which of the following statements regarding pigmented villonodular synovitis (PVNS) is true?
    a) Erosions are common in the hip.
    b) PVNS may have an association with trauma.
    c) Chromosomal abnormalities may exist.
    d) All of the above are true.
    e) None of the above is true.

The correct answer is (**d**). Erosive changes with PVNS are more frequent in less spacious joints, particularly the hip, shoulder, elbow, and ankle. A prior history of trauma has been reported in ~50% of patients. Variable chromosomal alterations have been described, strongly supporting the hypothesis that PVNS has a neoplastic origin.

2. Radionuclide three-phase bone scan findings of PVNS include which of the following?
    a) Increased uptake on delayed and blood flow phases
    b) Increased uptake on all three phases
    c) Increased uptake on blood pool and blood flow phases
    d) Negative uptake on all three phases
    e) None of the above

The correct answer is (**c**). Hypervascularity is typical of PVNS. This accounts for increased radionuclide uptake on the blood flow and blood pool images of the three-phase bone scan. Additionally, PVNS shows hypermetabolic activity on positron emission tomography/CT imaging.

■ **Case 86**

1. Boundaries of the quadrilateral space include which of the following?
   a) Teres minor
   b) Teres major
   c) Long head of the triceps
   d) Surgical neck of the humerus
   e) All of the above

The correct answer is (**e**). The quadrilateral space is positioned along the posterior and inferior margin of the glenohumeral joint. The superior border of the space is composed of the teres minor muscle. The inferior border is represented by the teres major muscle. The lateral margin is composed of the surgical neck of the humerus. The medial margin is made up of the long head of the triceps.

2. All of the following may serve as causes of quadrilateral space syndrome, except…
   a) Labral cysts
   b) Glenoid fractures
   c) Clavicle fractures
   d) Posterior shoulder dislocation

The correct answer is (**c**). The quadrilateral space is a relatively fixed anatomic region of the shoulder girdle which is particularly prone to injury. Large posterior and inferior paralabral cysts may extend into this region, causing mass effect upon the axillary nerve. Any fracture involving the surgical neck of the humerus or lateral scapula predisposes to this syndrome. Clavicular fractures are not associated with this syndrome given the distal location of the clavicle relative to the quadrilateral space. Glenohumeral subluxations/dislocations, local tumors, and arthroscopic interventions are additional causes of quadrilateral space syndrome.

■ **Case 87**

1. Impingement and/or snapping around the hip joint may implicate which of the following structures?
   a) Quadratus femoris
   b) Iliotibial band
   c) Iliopsoas tendon
   d) Gluteus maximus tendon
   e) All of the above

The correct answer is (**e**). Multiple variations of impingement and snapping exist in and around the hip joint. The quadratus femoris has been implicated in ischiofemoral impingement, with MR imaging demonstrating edema and/or atrophy within this muscle adjacent to the ischial tuberosity secondary to a narrowed ischiofemoral interval. The iliotibial band and gluteus maximus may serve as a source of external snapping around the hip. The posterior tensor fascia lata and the gluteus maximus may snap over the greater trochanter with various forms of hip flexion and extension. The iliopsoas tendon is implicated in the internal snapping hip with snapping of this tendon over the iliopectineal eminence with provocative maneuvers.

2. Which of the following represents characteristics of labral tearing at the hip?
   a) Shallow linear signal increase along the superior quadrant of the labral base at the junction with the hyaline cartilage
   b) Irregular signal increase extending through the majority of the labral base
   c) Fluid signal intensity extending between the peripheral labral margin and the joint capsule
   d) Contrast imbibition or fluid signal intensity extending through the entire labral base
   e) Both b and d

The correct answer is (**e**). MR arthrography enables optimal evaluation of the labrum of the hip. Arthrography is performed with a dilute gadolinium intra-articular injection ranging in volume between 15 and 20 mL. A normal labral sulcus may be encountered between the acetabular hyaline cartilage and the base of the labrum. This sulcus is shallow and smooth and is most commonly located along the anterior superior and posterior superior margins of the labrum. A normal capsular labral recess exists between the capsular insertion onto the acetabulum and the peripheral margin of the labrum. Fluid from a joint effusion or injected gadolinium solution may fill this normal recess and should not be confused with a labral tear. Labral tears have irregular edges and intrinsic MR signal abnormality extending partially or fully through the labral tissue and/or base of the labrum at the acetabular attachment. Anterior superior labral tears are fairly common. Posterior labral tears may be seen in young patients with a history of dysplasia or prior posterior hip dislocation. Cartilage fissuring and cystic bony changes may be seen adjacent to labral tears related to femoral acetabular impingement. Additionally, paralabral cysts frequently coexist with labral tears.

■ **Case 88**

1. Which of the following MRI findings is the best discriminator between osteomyelitis and Charcot arthropathy?
   a) Increased T2 bone marrow signal on fluid-sensitive MR images
   b) Focal fluid collection adjacent to bony structures demonstrating bone marrow edema
   c) Skin ulceration with adjacent bone marrow demonstrating a "ghost sign" on MRI
   d) Post-gadolinium enhancement of bone marrow
   e) None of the above

The correct answer is (**c**). Nearly all diabetic foot infections are related to contiguous spread of infection from a skin ulcer. Profound decreased T1 signal on fat-sensitive MR imaging which is contiguous with an ulceration or sinus tract is diagnostic of osteomyelitis. The "ghost sign" has been assigned to the T1 marrow signal changes. This sign is represented by nonvisualization of the infected bony structure on fat-sensitive T1 sequences secondary to replacement of the bone marrow by the infectious/inflammatory changes of osteomyelitis. The infected bone reappears with gadolinium-enhanced imaging and/or fat-sensitive T2-weighted imaging. Both osteomyelitis and Charcot arthropathy may demonstrate T2 bone marrow edema and enhancement. Fluid collections may be seen with both disease processes in the form of an abscess with osteomyelitis and a joint effusion with Charcot arthropathy. MR signal changes centered at an articulation favor Charcot arthropathy because this is a joint-centered process.

2. Which of the following radiographic features is characteristic of the diabetic foot?
   a) Avulsion fracture through the calcaneal tuberosity
   b) Talar dome osteochondral lesions
   c) Peroneal retinacular avulsions
   d) Medial clear space widening
   e) Both a and c

The correct answer is (**a**). An atraumatic Lisfranc fracture/dislocation is frequently associated with the diabetic foot secondary to Charcot arthropathy. Other radiographic findings characteristically seen in the diabetic foot include pedal vascular calcifications, diffuse soft tissue swelling, osteopenia, scattered foot ulcerations, midfoot collapse with a rocker-bottom foot deformity, nontraumatic avulsion fractures through the calcaneal tuberosity, and second metatarsal head and neck fractures. All of these findings are a direct or indirect result of diabetic neuropathy.

■ **Case 89**

1. MRI features of osteoid osteoma include which of the following?
   a) Low signal on all sequences with minimal enhancement
   b) Intense enhancement related to underlying hypervascularity
   c) Blooming artifact related to hemosiderin
   d) Hypointense T1 and hyperintense T2 signal
   e) None of the above

The correct answer is (**b**). The MR appearance of osteoid osteomas is variable. However, the typical nidus exhibits intermediate to decreased T1-weighted signal with heterogeneously increased T2 signal. Calcification within the nidus results in a signal void on both T1- and T2-weighted images. The enhancement pattern is typically diffuse and is related to the hypervascularity of this tumor. The hypervascular nature of osteoid osteomas is responsible for the extensive periosteal reaction. Perilesional soft tissue edema and enhancement may also be seen.

2. Which of the following features differentiates osteoid osteoma from osteoblastoma?
   a) Osteoblastoma is larger in size than osteoid osteoma.
   b) Osteoid osteoma may enlarge over time.
   c) Osteoid osteoma may exhibit fluid–fluid levels on MRI.
   d) Both a and c
   e) None of the above

The correct answer is (**a**). Osteoid osteoma and osteoblastoma share many similar imaging and histopathologic characteristics. However, osteoblastomas are typically larger in size containing a nidus measuring 1.5 to 2.0 cm with less surrounding sclerosis. Osteoblastoma is a less painful lesion and does not respond to NSAIDs as effectively as osteoid osteomas. Osteoblastoma has the potential to grow over time and may subsequently exhibit hemorrhagic fluid–fluid levels on MR imaging. Osteoid osteomas typically do not enlarge over time. Osteoblastomas may affect both the axial and appendicular skeleton, whereas osteoid osteomas typically affect the appendicular skeleton.

■ **Case 90**

1. Which of the following MRI features most reliably distinguishes reactive bone marrow edema from osteomyelitis in patients with septic arthritis?
   a) Extent of cartilage loss
   b) Subcortical depth and distribution of bone marrow signal abnormality
   c) Size of joint effusion
   d) Extent of synovial thickening
   e) Bone marrow T2 signal intensity

The correct answer is (**b**). Coexisting osteomyelitis in the setting of septic arthritis may be difficult to determine because septic arthritis frequently causes reactive bone marrow edema changes. However, the bone marrow edema pattern seen with osteomyelitis is typically more diffuse and multifocal, extending well beyond the subarticular cortical margins. Additionally, profoundly decreased T1 fat signal intensity has a strong association with osteomyelitis. Extent of cartilage loss, size of joint effusion, extent of synovial thickening, and intensity of T2 signal changes in the bone marrow offer little or no assistance in the diagnosis of osteomyelitis.

2. Phemister's triad is represented by which of the following?
    a) Rapid bone destruction, osteopenia, and bony debris
    b) Large joint effusion, periarticular osteopenia, and subchondral bone plate collapse
    c) Periarticular osteopenia, periarticular erosions, and gradual joint space loss
    d) Cystic bony resorption, osteopenia, and subluxation
    e) None of the above

The correct answer is (**c**). Phemister's triad is defined as juxta-articular osteopenia with peripheral bony erosions and gradual narrowing of the joint space. These are findings described with tuberculous arthritis. This granulomatous infection is more indolent in nature, resulting in less rapid and uniform joint space loss.

■ Case 91

1. In addition to erosive osteoarthritis, all of the following disease processes may involve the distal interphalangeal (DIP) joints of the hand except…
    a) Psoriatic arthritis
    b) Osteoarthritis
    c) Calcium pyrophosphate dihydrate disease (CPPD) arthropathy
    d) Multicentric reticulohistiocytosis
    e) All of the above

The correct answer is (**c**). Psoriatic arthritis represents a seronegative spondyloarthropathy with characteristic hand radiographic findings of a sausage digit and periarticular erosions admixed with bone proliferation involving the proximal and DIP joints. Osteoarthritis represents a degenerative process that typically affects the DIP joints, more commonly seen in females. CPPD represents a crystalline arthropathy. The hallmark findings of this arthropathy in the hand include hooklike osteophytes and erosive changes involving the second and third metacarpal heads with sparing of the interphalangeal joints. Multicentric reticulohistiocytosis is a systemic granulomatous disease typically affecting middle-aged females. This disease process is notorious for causing circumscribed or etched out erosions along the margins of the DIP joints.

2. Which of the following features helps in distinguishing between erosive and nonerosive osteoarthritis in the hands?
    a) Synovial inflammation
    b) Clinical presentation
    c) Joint distribution
    d) All of the above
    e) None of the above

The correct answer is (**d**). Erosive osteoarthritis represents an idiopathic variant of osteoarthritis. Whereas synovitis has been described with nonerosive osteoarthritis, a more prominent component of synovial inflammation is seen with erosive osteoarthritis, resulting in the central subarticular erosions. As a result of this synovial inflammation, these patients will present with polyarticular swelling, edema, tenderness, and erythema in contrast to complaints of localized pain as seen with nonerosive osteoarthritis. Nonerosive osteoarthritis is typically localized to the DIP joints. Erosive osteoarthritis may involve both the distal and proximal interphalangeal joints.

■ Case 92

1. Which of the following statements regarding the development of the tibial tuberosity is true?
    a) This ossification center represents an extension of the tibial epiphyseal cartilage.
    b) This structure contains fibrocartilage that eventually differentiates into bone.
    c) Inherent weakening of the tibial tuberosity occurs during its maturation.
    d) All of the above are true.
    e) None of the above is true.

The correct answer is (**d**). The tibial tuberosity apophysis represents an extension of the tibial epiphyseal cartilage. As this ossification center matures from fibrocartilage to bone, intermediate development of columnar cartilage occurs, causing weakening at this site. Completion of this entire maturation process may occur anywhere between 13 and 18 years of age.

2. A distinguishing feature of an acute tibial tuberosity apophyseal fracture from Osgood–Schlatter disease is which of the following?
    a) Soft tissue swelling
    b) Patella alta
    c) Tibial tuberosity fragmentation
    d) Tibial tuberosity fragmentation and displacement which involves the tibial epiphysis
    e) None of the above

The correct answer is (**d**). Osgood–Schlatter disease may predispose to development of acute tibial tuberosity avulsion fractures. These fractures are fairly common in teenage boys. Oblique radiographic positioning of the knee profiles the tibial tuberosity, enabling identification of acute fracture margins. Radiographic findings of distraction of the entire tibial tuberosity with extension into the tibial epiphysis and joint space are also consistent with this acute injury.

■ Case 93

1. Regarding assessment of the cervical prevertebral soft tissues, which of the following is true?
   a) Greater than 5 mm thickening at any level is abnormal.
   b) Marked variation in thickness most commonly occurs at C7.
   c) The C2 prevertebral soft tissues are considered abnormal if thicker than 10 mm.
   d) The C7 prevertebral soft tissues are considered abnormal if thicker than 10 mm.
   e) None of the above is true.

The correct answer is (**c**). Fullness of the cervical prevertebral soft tissues may serve as an important surrogate marker for underlying inflammation, neoplasm, hemorrhage, ligamentous injury, and occult fractures. Much variation exists in the normal prevertebral cervical soft tissue thickness throughout the human population. This is particularly true at the C4 level secondary to the underlying variable anatomy of the esophagus and larynx. As a rule of thumb, the upper limit of normal for prevertebral soft tissue thickness at the C2 vertebral body level should equal ~7 mm, whereas the upper limit of normal thickness at the C7 level should equal ~2 cm. A normal transition in thickness is typically seen at the C4 level.

2. Direct hematogenous spread of pathogens to the vertebral body occurs by which of the following routes?
   a) Vertebral body nutrient arterioles
   b) Batson's plexus
   c) Superior vena cava
   d) Both a and b
   e) None of the above

The correct answer is (**d**). Bloodborne pathogens are capable of directly inoculating the vertebral body by antegrade flow through the nutrient arterioles of the vertebral bodies. These arterioles are more numerous along the anterior aspect of the vertebral body, which usually represents the initial site of involvement as detected on radiography. From this site, the infection may spread to the remaining vertebral body along the medullary space. Retrograde blood flow through the valveless Batson's venous plexus serves as one of the primary causes for vertebral body metastases. This valveless plexus also enables hematogenous pathogens direct access to the vertebral bodies. The superior vena cava does not serve as a direct route for pathogens to infiltrate the vertebral bodies.

■ Case 94

1. Complications of osteochondroma include which of the following?
   a) Fracture
   b) Adventitial bursal formation
   c) Vascular/neural impingement
   d) Sarcomatous degeneration
   e) All of the above

The correct answer is (**e**). The majority of osteochondromas will cause no complications. However, traumatic fractures through osteochondromas have been reported. Development of an adventitial bursa may occur between the cartilaginous cap/bony protuberance and overlying ligamentous, tendinous, and osseous structures. This results in focal soft tissue fullness. This is commonly seen with ventral scapular body osteochondromas. Other potential complications include bony impingement into the spinal cord, peripheral nerves, or vascular structures. The most serious complication of osteochondroma is secondary degeneration into a chondrosarcoma, seen in ~1% of solitary osteochondromas.

2. Which of the following statements is true?
   a) Osteochondromas may occur secondary to childhood irradiation.
   b) The pes anserine spur represents a variant of osteochondroma.
   c) Subungual exostoses share the same pathogenesis as osteochondroma.
   d) All of the above are true.
   e) None of the above is true.

The correct answer is (**a**). Osteochondroma represents the most common benign radiation-induced tumor. This is typically seen in patients irradiated between the ages of 8 months and 11 years and is believed to be related to injury of the epiphyseal plate allowing for abnormal cartilage migration into the metaphysis. The prevalence of osteochondromas in this subset of patients ranges from 6 to 25%. The pes anserine spur is a bony prominence, pointed away from the knee joint, arising from the proximal medial tibial metaphysis. This structure does not contain a cartilaginous cap and therefore does not represent a true osteochondroma. A subungual exostosis most commonly arises from the dorsal medial aspect of the great toe distal phalanx, deep to the nailbed. This lesion shows no corticomedullary continuity with the underlying bone. Although this lesion contains a fibrocartilaginous cap, its etiology has been linked to repetitive trauma and/or chronic inflammation/infection.

■ Case 95

1. Which of the following MR characteristics enable differentiation of recurrent myxoid liposarcoma from a seroma?
   a) T1 signal characteristics
   b) T2 signal characteristics
   c) Enhancement pattern
   d) Location
   e) None of the above

The correct answer is (**c**). Postoperative seromas and recurrent myxoid liposarcoma both appear as cystic lesions on nonenhanced MRI with decreased T1 and increased T2 signal. However, tumor recurrence typically reveals post-gadolinium enhancement, whereas a seroma will not enhance.

2. Described patterns of enhancement in myxoid liposarcoma include all of the following except...
   a) Rim enhancement
   b) Absence of enhancement
   c) Diffuse heterogeneous enhancement
   d) Diffuse homogeneous enhancement

The correct answer is (**a**). The enhancement pattern plays a crucial role in evaluation and diagnosis of myxoid liposarcoma. Described enhancement patterns depend upon the level of cellularity and vascularity along with the presence or absence of intratumoral necrosis. Myxoid liposarcomas with a prominent arborizing capillary pattern and abundant myxoid matrix with hypercellularity demonstrate profound homogeneous enhancement. Variants of this tumor type may demonstrate a focal compact region of hypercellularity, hypervascularity, and myxoid matrix admixed with necrosis and hemorrhage, resulting in a heterogeneous enhancement pattern. Myxoid liposarcomas may be highly necrotic and hypocellular, with an abundance of mucinous debris exhibiting no enhancement. A rim enhancement pattern is not typical for this neoplasm.

■ Case 96

1. Which of the following are predisposing factors for periprosthetic fractures?
   a) Postmenopausal osteoporosis
   b) Stress shielding
   c) Osteolysis
   d) All of the above
   e) None of the above

The correct answer is (**d**). Any process that diminishes bone stock around hip arthroplasty components increases the risk for a periprosthetic fracture. Postmenopausal osteoporosis, bone resorption from stress shielding, and osteolysis represent such risk factors.

2. CT imaging of joint arthroplasty is most compromised by which of the following?
   a) Volume averaging
   b) Beam hardening
   c) Composition of polyethylene components
   d) All of the above
   e) None of the above

The correct answer is (**b**). Metallic components used for arthroplasty or fracture fixation result in photon starvation and beam hardening with CT imaging. The metallic components attenuate the low-energy photons, shifting the spectrum toward high-energy photons and diminishing the diagnostic capability. Increasing the peak kilovoltage may overcome this obstacle. Increasing tube current will also reduce photon starvation. These techniques may be utilized in an effort to improve diagnostic capability. Polyethylene components have minimal effect on CT image quality. Volume averaging is not a recognized obstacle in the CT evaluation of arthroplasties.

■ Case 97

1. All of the following have an increased risk of chondrosarcomatous degeneration, except...
   a) Ollier disease
   b) Maffucci syndrome
   c) Osteopoikilosis
   d) Enchondroma
   e) Osteochondroma

The correct answer is (**c**). Secondary chondrosarcoma is a diagnosis used to describe the development of chondrosarcoma from an underlying benign bony lesion. The solitary enchondroma and osteochondroma have little malignant potential with an overall reported risk of < 1% chance of malignant transformation to chondrosarcoma. Multiple hereditary exostosis carries a slightly increased risk of malignant degeneration ranging between 2 and 5%. Multiple enchondromas may exist in a condition referred to as Ollier disease. When this condition is associated with soft tissue hemangiomas, the designation of Maffucci syndrome is used. Both of these conditions are congenital and carry a 30 to 50% increased risk of chondrosarcomatous degeneration, particularly Maffucci syndrome. Osteopoikilosis represents a bone-forming dystrophy manifested by multiple periarticular bone islands and has no malignant potential.

2. Which of the following radiographic features favor malignant degeneration of an osteochondroma to a chondrosarcoma?
    a) Minimal lesion enlargement during the first decade of life
    b) Progression of chondroid calcifications following skeletal maturity
    c) Pedunculated morphology
    d) Sessile morphology
    e) None of the above

The correct answer is (**b**). The radiographic appearance of an osteochondroma should stabilize at skeletal maturity. Conversion of an osteochondroma to a secondary chondrosarcoma may be represented by any change in lesion size after this point in time. Other worrisome findings include osteolysis or an irregular and indistinct appearance involving the bony component of the lesion. Development of a large soft tissue mass along with an increase in chondroid calcifications suggests malignant degeneration. The sessile or pedunculated nature of osteochondroma has no association with malignant potential.

■ **Case 98**

1. Causes of Achilles tendon pathology include which of the following?
    a) Anabolic steroid use
    b) Xanthomatosis
    c) Fluoroquinolones
    d) All of the above
    e) None of the above

The correct answer is (**d**). Although the most common cause of Achilles tendon pathology is related to traumatic injury and overuse, other conditions are associated with pathology at this site. Anabolic steroid abuse has been linked to connective tissue and collagen dysfunction within tendons resulting in alteration of tensile strength and tendon rupture. Xanthomatosis represents an inherited metabolic disease which causes focal thickening of the Achilles tendon secondary to intrasubstance xanthomas which may mimic Achilles tendinopathy. Fluoroquinolone antibiotic use may result in an inflammatory response within the Achilles tendon that is similar to that observed in overuse syndromes.

2. Regarding Achilles tendon anatomy, which of the following is true?
    a) The Achilles tendon does not contain a synovial lining.
    b) The pre-Achilles fat provides no function to the Achilles tendon.
    c) No bursae are associated with the Achilles tendon.
    d) All of the above are true.
    e) None of the above is true.

The correct answer is (**a**). A paratenon surrounds the Achilles tendon, as opposed to a tendon sheath. The paratenon is a filmy membrane allowing gliding of the Achilles tendon with flexion and extension. The pre-Achilles fat, or Kager's fat pad, represents a triangle of fatty tissue deep to the Achilles tendon. This fat pad structurally supports blood supply to the Achilles tendon and may provide a mechanical advantage to the active flexion and extension of the Achilles. Two separate bursae are located along the distal Achilles tendon, the retrocalcaneal and retro-Achilles bursae. The retrocalcaneal bursa, located between the Achilles tendon and posterior superior calcaneus, represents a true bursa which may contain up to 3 mm of fluid in the normal setting. Haglund's deformity and seronegative spondyloarthropathies may cause bursitis at this level. A potential retro-Achilles adventitial bursa may be present superficial to the posterior Achilles tendon at the level of the calcaneal insertion. Under normal circumstances, no fluid is seen at this site.

■ **Case 99**

1. Regarding peroneal tendon anatomy, which of the following is true?
    a) The peroneal tendons share a common tendon sheath distal to the lateral malleolus.
    b) The peroneus brevis tendon is lateral to the peroneus longus tendon at the level of the lateral malleolus.
    c) The peroneus brevis tendon inserts at the base of the fifth metatarsal.
    d) The peroneus longus tendon inserts at the base of the fifth metatarsal.
    e) None of the above is true.

The correct answer is (**c**). The peroneal tendons share a common tendon sheath posterior to the lateral malleolus where the peroneus brevis is typically positioned anterior and medial to the peroneus longus. The peroneus longus tendon inserts at the level of the plantar medial cuneiform and proximal first metatarsal. The peroneus brevis inserts onto the lateral base of the fifth metatarsal.

2. Which of the following represents peroneal muscle tendon variants?
    a) Peroneus digiti minimi
    b) Peroneus accessories
    c) Peroneus digiti quinti
    d) Peroneus calcaneus externum
    e) All of the above

The correct answer is (**e**). Multiple accessory peroneal muscles have been described. The incidence of these accessory muscles is variable and much confusion exists regarding their terminology. These variants include the peroneus digiti minimi, peroneus accessories, peroneus digiti quinti, and peroneus calcaneus externum. Variable origins and insertions of these structures have been described.

■ Case 100

1. The MRI features of a meniscal ossicle are easily identified on which of the following sequences?
   a) Short tau inversion recovery (STIR)
   b) T2-weighted imaging with fat saturation
   c) T1-weighted imaging without fat saturation
   d) Post-gadolinium T1-weighted fat-suppressed imaging
   e) None of the above

The correct answer is (**c**). An abundance of fat is present within the meniscal ossicle. This enables adequate identification on MR sequences which are fat sensitive. STIR and fat-suppressed imaging sequences are not fat sensitive and limit visualization of this structure.

2. Regarding meniscal ossicles, which of the following is false?
   a) Exists as a normal variant in domestic cats, rodents, and tigers
   b) May occur as a result of crystalline deposition
   c) Occurs in the posterior horn of the medial meniscus, in part, as a result of the abundant vascularity
   d) May serve as a source of intermittent pain
   e) All of the above

The correct answer is (**b**). Ossification within the meniscus has no association with crystalline deposits. Proposed theories are posttraumatic metaplasia or heterotopic ossification. The meniscal ossicle has been identified in other species. The abundance of geniculate vascularity in the posterior horn medial meniscus has been suggested as a potential predisposing factor for meniscal ossification in this region. Occasionally, patients may complain of pain related to the meniscal ossicle.

Further Readings

Case 1

Porrino JA Jr, Kohl CA, Taljanovic M, Rogers LF. Diagnosis of proximal femoral insufficiency fractures in patients receiving bisphosphonate therapy. AJR Am J Roentgenol 2010;194(4):1061–1064

Case 2

Boyse TD, Fessell DP, Jacobson JA, Lin J, van Holsbeeck MT, Hayes CW. US of soft-tissue foreign bodies and associated complications with surgical correlation. Radiographics 2001;21(5):1251–1256

Case 3

Park JS, Ryu KN, Yoon KH. Meniscal flounce on knee MRI: correlation with meniscal locations after positional changes. AJR Am J Roentgenol 2006;187(2):364–370

Case 4

Cerezal L, Abascal F, García-Valtuille R, Del Piñal F. Wrist MR arthrography: how, why, when. Radiol Clin North Am 2005;43(4):709–731, viii

Case 5

McDonald ES, Yi ES, Wenger DE. Best cases from the AFIP: extraabdominal desmoid-type fibromatosis. Radiographics 2008;28(3):901–906

Case 6

Murphey MD, Sartoris DJ, Quale JL, Pathria MN, Martin NL. Musculoskeletal manifestations of chronic renal insufficiency. Radiographics 1993;13(2):357–379

Case 7

Dillenseger JP, Molière S, Choquet P, Goetz C, Ehlinger M, Bierry G. An illustrative review to understand and manage metal-induced artifacts in musculoskeletal MRI: a primer and updates. Skeletal Radiol 2016;45(5):677–688

Fritz J, Lurie B, Miller TT, Potter HG. MR imaging of hip arthroplasty implants. Radiographics 2014;34(4): E106–E132

Case 8

Kassarjian A, Tomas X, Cerezal L, Canga A, Llopis E. MRI of the quadratus femoris muscle: anatomic considerations and pathologic lesions. AJR Am J Roentgenol 2011;197(1):170–174

Case 9

Bradley DM, Bergman AG, Dillingham MF. MR imaging of cyclops lesions. AJR Am J Roentgenol 2000;174(3):719–726

Case 10

Nakata W, Katou S, Fujita A, Nakata M, Lefor AT, Sugimoto H. Biceps pulley: normal anatomy and associated lesions at MR arthrography. Radiographics 2011;31(3):791–810

Petchprapa CN, Beltran LS, Jazrawi LM, Kwon YW, Babb JS, Recht MP. The rotator interval: a review of anatomy, function, and normal and abnormal MRI appearance. AJR Am J Roentgenol 2010;195(3):567–576

Case 11

Jacobson JA, Girish G, Jiang Y, Resnick D. Radiographic evaluation of arthritis: inflammatory conditions. Radiology 2008;248(2):378–389

Hermann KG, Althoff CE, Schneider U, et al. Spinal changes in patients with spondyloarthritis: comparison of MR imaging and radiographic appearances. Radiographics 2005;25(3):559–569, discussion 569–570

Case 12

Girish G, Glazebrook KN, Jacobson JA. Advanced imaging in gout. AJR Am J Roentgenol 2013;201(3):515–525

Jacobson JA, Girish G, Jiang Y, Sabb BJ. Radiographic evaluation of arthritis: degenerative joint disease and variations. Radiology 2008;248(3):737–747

Monu JUV, Pope TL Jr. Gout: a clinical and radiologic review. Radiol Clin North Am 2004;42(1):169–184

■ **Case 13**

Rosenberg ZS, Bencardino J, Astion D, Schweitzer ME, Rokito A, Sheskier S. MRI features of chronic injuries of the superior peroneal retinaculum. AJR Am J Roentgenol 2003;181(6):1551–1557

■ **Case 14**

Bancroft LW, Blankenbaker DG. Imaging of the tendons about the pelvis. AJR Am J Roentgenol 2010;195(3):605–617

Yukata K, Nakai S, Goto T, et al. Cystic lesion around the hip joint. World J Orthop 2015;6(9):688–704

■ **Case 15**

Parellada AJ, Gopez AG, Morrison WB, et al. Distal intersection tenosynovitis of the wrist: a lesser-known extensor tendinopathy with characteristic MR imaging features. Skeletal Radiol 2007;36(3):203–208

■ **Case 16**

Cockenpot E, Lefebvre G, Demondion X, Chantelot C, Cotten A. Imaging of sports-related hand and wrist injuries: sports imaging series 1. Radiology 2016;279(3):674–692

Conway WF, Destouet JM, Gilula LA, Bellinghausen HW, Weeks PM. The carpal boss: an overview of radiographic evaluation. Radiology 1985;156(1):29–31

■ **Case 17**

Costello RF, Beall DP, Van Zandt BL, Stapp AM, Martin HD, Steury SW. Contrast reaction from hip arthrogram. Emerg Radiol. 2007;14(1):59–61

Shahid M, Shyamsundar S, Bali N, McBryde C, O'Hara J, Bache E. Efficacy of using an air arthrogram for EUA and injection of the hip joint in adults. J Orthop. 2014; 11(3):132–135.

■ **Case 18**

Garcia GM, McCord GC, Kumar R. Hydroxyapatite crystal deposition disease. Semin Musculoskelet Radiol 2003;7(3):187–193

Steinbach LS. Calcium pyrophosphate dihydrate and calcium hydroxyapatite crystal deposition diseases: imaging perspectives. Radiol Clin North Am 2004;42(1):185–205, vii

■ **Case 19**

Walz DM, Newman JS, Konin GP, Ross G. Epicondylitis: pathogenesis, imaging, and treatment. Radiographics 2010;30(1):167–184

■ **Case 20**

Beltran J, Rosenberg ZS, Chandnani VP, Cuomo F, Beltran S, Rokito A. Glenohumeral instability: evaluation with MR arthrography. Radiographics 1997;17(3):657–673

■ **Case 21**

Dinauer PA, Brixey CJ, Moncur JT, Fanburg-Smith JC, Murphey MD. Pathologic and MR imaging features of benign fibrous soft-tissue tumors in adults. Radiographics 2007;27(1):173–187

Ochsner JE, Sewall SA, Brooks GN, Agni R. Best cases from the AFIP: Elastofibroma dorsi. Radiographics 2006;26(6):1873–1876

■ **Case 22**

Nguyen JC, De Smet AA, Graf BK, Rosas HG. MR imaging-based diagnosis and classification of meniscal tears. Radiographics 2014;34(4):981–999

■ **Case 23**

Clavero JA, Alomar X, Monill JM, et al. MR imaging of ligament and tendon injuries of the fingers. Radiographics 2002;22(2):237–256

Hinke DH, Erickson SJ, Chamoy L, Timins ME. Ulnar collateral ligament of the thumb: MR findings in cadavers, volunteers, and patients with ligamentous injury (gamekeeper's thumb). AJR Am J Roentgenol 1994;163(6):1431–1434

■ **Case 24**

Alyas F, Curtis M, Speed C, Saifuddin A, Connell D. MR imaging appearances of acromioclavicular joint dislocation. Radiographics 2008;28(2):463–479, quiz 619

Antonio GE, Cho JH, Chung CB, Trudell DJ, Resnick D. Pictorial essay. MR imaging appearance and classification of acromioclavicular joint injury. AJR Am J Roentgenol 2003;180(4):1103–1110

■ Case 25

Koulouris G, Connell D. Hamstring muscle complex: an imaging review. Radiographics 2005;25(3):571–586

Rubin DA. Imaging diagnosis and prognostication of hamstring injuries. AJR Am J Roentgenol 2012;199(3):525–533

■ Case 26

Ahn KS, Kang CH, Oh YW, Jeong WK. Correlation between magnetic resonance imaging and clinical impairment in patients with adhesive capsulitis. Skeletal Radiol 2012;41(10):1301–1308

Petchprapa CN, Beltran LS, Jazrawi LM, Kwon YW, Babb JS, Recht MP. The rotator interval: a review of anatomy, function, and normal and abnormal MRI appearance. AJR Am J Roentgenol 2010;195(3):567–576

■ Case 27

Rosenberg ZS, Beltran J, Bencardino JT. MR imaging of the ankle and foot. Radiographics 2000;20(Spec No):S153–S179

Schweitzer ME, Karasick D. MR imaging of disorders of the posterior tibialis tendon. AJR Am J Roentgenol 2000;175(3):627–635

■ Case 28

Rana RS, Wu JS, Eisenberg RL. Periosteal reaction. AJR Am J Roentgenol 2009;193(4):W259-W272

■ Case 29

Anderson SE, Steinbach LS, De Monaco D, Bonel HM, Hurtienne Y, Voegelin E. "Baby wrist": MRI of an overuse syndrome in mothers. AJR Am J Roentgenol 2004;182(3):719–724

Glajchen N, Schweitzer M. MRI features in de Quervain's tenosynovitis of the wrist. Skeletal Radiol 1996;25(1):63–65

■ Case 30

Lawrence DA, Rolen MF, Haims AH, Zayour Z, Moukaddam HA. Tarsal coalitions: radiographic, CT, and MR imaging findings. HSS J 2014;10(2):153–166

Newman JS, Newberg AH. Congenital tarsal coalition: multimodality evaluation with emphasis on CT and MR imaging. Radiographics 2000;20(2):321–332, quiz 526–527, 532

■ Case 31

Bergin D, Morrison WB, Carrino JA, Nallamshetty SN, Bartolozzi AR. Anterior cruciate ligament ganglia and mucoid degeneration: coexistence and clinical correlation. AJR Am J Roentgenol 2004;182(5):1283–1287

Papadopoulou P. The celery stalk sign. Radiology 2007;245(3):916–917

■ Case 32

Frick MA, Collins MS, Adkins MC. Postoperative imaging of the knee. Radiol Clin North Am 2006;44(3):367–389

Mulcahy H, Chew FS. Current concepts in knee replacement: complications. AJR Am J Roentgenol 2014;202(1):W76-86

■ Case 33

Hunter TB, Peltier LF, Lund PJ. Radiologic history exhibit. Musculoskeletal eponyms: who are those guys? Radiographics 2000;20(3):819–836

Mulligan ME. Ankle and foot trauma. Semin Musculoskelet Radiol 2000;4(2):241–253

Siddiqui NA, Galizia MS, Almusa E, Omar IM. Evaluation of the tarsometatarsal joint using conventional radiography, CT, and MR imaging. Radiographics 2014;34(2):514–531

■ Case 34

Douis H, Saifuddin A. The imaging of cartilaginous bone tumours. I. Benign lesions. Skeletal Radiol 2012;41(10):1195–1212

Robbin MR, Murphey MD. Benign chondroid neoplasms of bone. Semin Musculoskelet Radiol 2000;4(1):45–58

■ Case 35

Jacobson JA. Shoulder US: anatomy, technique, and scanning pitfalls. Radiology 2011;260(1):6–16

■ **Case 36**

Parman LM, Murphey MD. Alphabet soup: cystic lesions of bone. Semin Musculoskelet Radiol 2000;4(1):89–101

■ **Case 37**

Boles CA, Martin DF. Synovial plicae in the knee. AJR Am J Roentgenol 2001;177(1):221–227

García-Valtuille R, Abascal F, Cerezal L, et al. Anatomy and MR imaging appearances of synovial plicae of the knee. Radiographics 2002;22(4):775–784

■ **Case 38**

Bencardino JT, Gyftopoulos S, Palmer WE. Imaging in anterior glenohumeral instability. Radiology 2013;269(2):323–337

Carlson CL. The "J" sign. Radiology 2004;232(3):725–726

■ **Case 39**

Goergen TG, Resnick D, Greenway G, Saltzstein SL. Dorsal defect of the patella (DDP): a characteristic radiographic lesion. Radiology 1979;130(2):333–336

van Holsbeeck M, Vandamme B, Marchal G, Martens M, Victor J, Baert AL. Dorsal defect of the patella: concept of its origin and relationship with bipartite and multipartite patella. Skeletal Radiol 1987;16(4):304–311

■ **Case 40**

Chakarun CJ, Forrester DM, Gottsegen CJ, Patel DB, White EA, Matcuk GR Jr. Giant cell tumor of bone: review, mimics, and new developments in treatment. Radiographics 2013;33(1):197–211

Murphey MD, Nomikos GC, Flemming DJ, Gannon FH, Temple HT, Kransdorf MJ. From the archives of AFIP. Imaging of giant cell tumor and giant cell reparative granuloma of bone: radiologic-pathologic correlation. Radiographics 2001;21(5):1283–1309

■ **Case 41**

Freire V, Guérini H, Campagna R, et al. Imaging of hand and wrist cysts: a clinical approach. AJR Am J Roentgenol 2012;199(5):W618–628

Jacobson JA. Musculoskeletal sonography and MR imaging. A role for both imaging methods. Radiol Clin North Am 1999;37(4):713–735

Oneson SR, Scales LM, Erickson SJ, Timins ME. MR imaging of the painful wrist. Radiographics 1996;16(5):997–1008

■ **Case 42**

Flores DV, Smitaman E, Huang BK, Resnick DL. Segond fracture: an MR evaluation of 146 patients with emphasis on the avulsed bone fragment and what attaches to it. Skeletal Radiol 2016;45(12):1635–1647

Porrino J Jr, Maloney E, Richardson M, Mulcahy H, Ha A, Chew FS. The anterolateral ligament of the knee: MRI appearance, association with the Segond fracture, and historical perspective. AJR Am J Roentgenol 2015;204(2):367–373

Stevens MA, El-Khoury GY, Kathol MH, Brandser EA, Chow S. Imaging features of avulsion injuries. Radiographics 1999;19(3):655–672

■ **Case 43**

Ihde LL, Forrester DM, Gottsegen CJ, et al. Sclerosing bone dysplasias: review and differentiation from other causes of osteosclerosis. Radiographics 2011;31(7):1865–1882

■ **Case 44**

Ashman CJ, Klecker RJ, Yu JS. Forefoot pain involving the metatarsal region: differential diagnosis with MR imaging. Radiographics 2001;21(6):1425–1440

Bencardino J, Rosenberg ZS, Beltran J, Liu X, Marty-Delfaut E. Morton's neuroma: is it always symptomatic? AJR Am J Roentgenol 2000;175(3):649–653

■ **Case 45**

Smith SE, Murphey MD, Motamedi K, Mulligan ME, Resnik CS, Gannon FH. From the archives of the AFIP. Radiologic spectrum of Paget disease of bone and its complications with pathologic correlation. Radiographics 2002;22(5):1191–1216

Theodorou DJ, Theodorou SJ, Kakitsubata Y. Imaging of Paget disease of bone and its musculoskeletal complications: review. AJR Am J Roentgenol 2011;196 (6, Suppl):S64–S75

■ Case 46

Blacksin MF, Ha DH, Hameed M, Aisner S. Superficial soft-tissue masses of the extremities. Radiographics 2006;26(5):1289–1304

Bonilla-Yoon I, Masih S, Patel DB, et al. The Morel-Lavallée lesion: pathophysiology, clinical presentation, imaging features, and treatment options. Emerg Radiol 2014;21(1):35–43

Mellado JM, Pérez del Palomar L, Díaz L, Ramos A, Saurí A. Long-standing Morel-Lavallée lesions of the trochanteric region and proximal thigh: MRI features in five patients. AJR Am J Roentgenol 2004;182(5):1289–1294

■ Case 47

Bencardino JT, Beltran J, Feldman MI, Rose DJ. MR imaging of complications of anterior cruciate ligament graft reconstruction. Radiographics 2009;29(7):2115–2126

Meyers AB, Haims AH, Menn K, Moukaddam H. Imaging of anterior cruciate ligament repair and its complications. AJR Am J Roentgenol 2010;194(2):476–484

■ Case 48

Murphey MD, Robbin MR, McRae GA, Flemming DJ, Temple HT, Kransdorf MJ. The many faces of osteosarcoma. Radiographics 1997;17(5):1205–1231

■ Case 49

Baek HJ, Lee SJ, Cho KH, et al. Subungual tumors: clinico-pathologic correlation with US and MR imaging findings. Radiographics 2010;30(6):1621–1636

Glazebrook KN, Laundre BJ, Schiefer TK, Inwards CY. Imaging features of glomus tumors. Skeletal Radiol 2011;40(7):855–862

■ Case 50

Ali S, Cunningham R, Amin M, Popoff SN, Mohamed F, Barbe MF. The extensor carpi ulnaris pseudolesion: evaluation with microCT, histology, and MRI. Skeletal Radiol 2015;44(12):1735–1743

Campbell D, Campbell R, O'Connor P, Hawkes R. Sports-related extensor carpi ulnaris pathology: a review of functional anatomy, sports injury and management. Br J Sports Med 2013;47(17):1105–1111

Vezeridis PS, Yoshioka H, Han R, Blazar P. Ulnar-sided wrist pain. Part I: anatomy and physical examination. Skeletal Radiol 2010;39(8):733–745

Watanabe A, Souza F, Vezeridis PS, Blazar P, Yoshioka H. Ulnar-sided wrist pain. II. Clinical imaging and treatment. Skeletal Radiol 2010;39(9):837–857

■ Case 51

Beck BR, Bergman AG, Miner M, et al. Tibial stress injury: relationship of radiographic, nuclear medicine bone scanning, MR imaging, and CT severity grades to clinical severity and time to healing. Radiology 2012;263(3):811–818

Kijowski R, Choi J, Shinki K, Del Rio AM, De Smet A. Validation of MRI classification system for tibial stress injuries. AJR Am J Roentgenol 2012;198(4):878–884

Spitz DJ, Newberg AH. Imaging of stress fractures in the athlete. Radiol Clin North Am 2002;40(2):313–331

■ Case 52

Gottsegen CJ, Eyer BA, White EA, Learch TJ, Forrester D. Avulsion fractures of the knee: imaging findings and clinical significance. Radiographics 2008;28(6):1755–1770

Strub WM. The arcuate sign. Radiology 2007;244(2):620–621

Vinson EN, Major NM, Helms CA. The posterolateral corner of the knee. AJR Am J Roentgenol 2008;190(2):449–458

■ Case 53

Jelinek JS, Murphey MD, Kransdorf MJ, Shmookler BM, Malawer MM, Hur RC. Parosteal osteosarcoma: value of MR imaging and CT in the prediction of histologic grade. Radiology 1996;201(3):837–842

Murphey MD, Robbin MR, McRae GA, Flemming DJ, Temple HT, Kransdorf MJ. The many faces of osteosarcoma. Radiographics 1997;17(5):1205–1231

White LM, Kandel R. Osteoid-producing tumors of bone. Semin Musculoskelet Radiol 2000;4(1):25–43

■ Case 54

Cerezal L, del Piñal F, Abascal F, García-Valtuille R, Pereda T, Canga A. Imaging findings in ulnar-sided wrist impaction syndromes. Radiographics 2002;22(1):105–121

Watanabe A, Souza F, Vezeridis PS, Blazar P, Yoshioka H. Ulnar-sided wrist pain. II. Clinical imaging and treatment. Skeletal Radiol 2010;39(9):837–857

■ **Case 55**

Bennett DL, Ohashi K, El-Khoury GY. Spondyloarthropathies: ankylosing spondylitis and psoriatic arthritis. Radiol Clin North Am 2004;42(1):121–134

Jacobson JA, Girish G, Jiang Y, Resnick D. Radiographic evaluation of arthritis: inflammatory conditions. Radiology 2008;248(2):378–389

Navallas M, Ares J, Beltrán B, Lisbona MP, Maymó J, Solano A. Sacroiliitis associated with axial spondyloarthropathy: new concepts and latest trends. Radiographics 2013;33(4):933–956

■ **Case 56**

Bencardino JT, Beltran J, Feldman MI, Rose DJ. MR imaging of complications of anterior cruciate ligament graft reconstruction. Radiographics 2009;29(7):2115–2126

Ghazikhanian V, Beltran J, Nikac V, Feldman M, Bencardino JT. Tibial tunnel and pretibial cysts following ACL graft reconstruction: MR imaging diagnosis. Skeletal Radiol 2012;41(11):1375–1379

■ **Case 57**

Mulcahy H, Chew FS. Current concepts of hip arthroplasty for radiologists: part 2, revisions and complications. AJR Am J Roentgenol 2012;199(3):570–580

Roth TD, Maertz NA, Parr JA, Buckwalter KA, Choplin RH. CT of the hip prosthesis: appearance of components, fixation, and complications. Radiographics 2012;32(4):1089–1107

■ **Case 58**

Flemming DJ, Murphey MD. Enchondroma and chondrosarcoma. Semin Musculoskelet Radiol 2000;4(1):59–71

Murphey MD, Flemming DJ, Boyea SR, Bojescul JA, Sweet DE, Temple HT. Enchondroma versus chondrosarcoma in the appendicular skeleton: differentiating features. Radiographics 1998;18(5):1213–1237, quiz 1244–1245

■ **Case 59**

Bancroft LW, Peterson JJ, Kransdorf MJ. Cysts, geodes, and erosions. Radiol Clin North Am 2004;42(1):73–87

Manaster BJ. From the RSNA refresher courses. Total hip arthroplasty: radiographic evaluation. Radiographics 1996;16(3):645–660

Mulcahy H, Chew FS. Current concepts of hip arthroplasty for radiologists: part 2, revisions and complications. AJR Am J Roentgenol 2012;199(3):570–580

Taljanovic MS, Jones MD, Hunter TB, et al. Joint arthroplasties and prostheses. Radiographics 2003;23(5):1295–1314

■ **Case 60**

McCarthy EF, Sundaram M. Heterotopic ossification: a review. Skeletal Radiol 2005;34(10):609–619

■ **Case 61**

Llauger J, Palmer J, Rosón N, Cremades R, Bagué S. Pigmented villonodular synovitis and giant cell tumors of the tendon sheath: radiologic and pathologic features. AJR Am J Roentgenol 1999;172(4):1087–1091

■ **Case 62**

Llauger J, Palmer J, Rosón N, Cremades R, Bagué S. Pigmented villonodular synovitis and giant cell tumors of the tendon sheath: radiologic and pathologic features. AJR Am J Roentgenol 1999;172(4):1087–1091

Murphey MD, Rhee JH, Lewis RB, Fanburg-Smith JC, Flemming DJ, Walker EA. Pigmented villonodular synovitis: radiologic-pathologic correlation. Radiographics 2008;28(5):1493–1518

Sheldon PJ, Forrester DM, Learch TJ. Imaging of intraarticular masses. Radiographics 2005;25(1):105–119

■ **Case 63**

Andreisek G, Crook DW, Burg D, Marincek B, Weishaupt D. Peripheral neuropathies of the median, radial, and ulnar nerves: MR imaging features. Radiographics 2006;26(5):1267–1287

Miller TT, Reinus WR. Nerve entrapment syndromes of the elbow, forearm, and wrist. AJR Am J Roentgenol 2010;195(3):585–594

■ Case 64

Morelli JN, Runge VM, Ai F, et al. An image-based approach to understanding the physics of MR artifacts. Radiographics 2011;31(3):849–866

Peh WC, Chan JH. Artifacts in musculoskeletal magnetic resonance imaging: identification and correction. Skeletal Radiol 2001;30(4):179–191

■ Case 65

Fitzpatrick KA, Taljanovic MS, Speer DP, et al. Imaging findings of fibrous dysplasia with histopathologic and intraoperative correlation. AJR Am J Roentgenol 2004;182(6):1389–1398

Miller SL, Hoffer FA. Malignant and benign bone tumors. Radiol Clin North Am 2001;39(4):673–699

Smith SE, Kransdorf MJ. Primary musculoskeletal tumors of fibrous origin. Semin Musculoskelet Radiol 2000;4(1):73–88

■ Case 66

Diederichs G, Issever AS, Scheffler S. MR imaging of patellar instability: injury patterns and assessment of risk factors. Radiographics 2010;30(4):961–981

■ Case 67

Jacobson JA, Girish G, Jiang Y, Resnick D. Radiographic evaluation of arthritis: inflammatory conditions. Radiology 2008;248(2):378–389

Sommer OJ, Kladosek A, Weiler V, Czembirek H, Boeck M, Stiskal M. Rheumatoid arthritis: a practical guide to state-of-the-art imaging, image interpretation, and clinical implications. Radiographics 2005;25(2):381–398

■ Case 68

Dwek JR. Clinical perspective. A structural and mechanism-based perspective toward understanding pediatric and adult sports injuries. AJR Am J Roentgenol 2016;206(5):980–986

Hunter TB, Peltier LF, Lund PJ. Radiologic history exhibit. Musculoskeletal eponyms: who are those guys? Radiographics 2000;20(3):819–836

Lee P, Hunter TB, Taljanovic M. Musculoskeletal colloquialisms: how did we come up with these names? Radiographics 2004;24(4):1009–1027

Stevens MA, El-Khoury GY, Kathol MH, Brandser EA, Chow S. Imaging features of avulsion injuries. Radiographics 1999;19(3):655–672

■ Case 69

Fayad LM, Kawamoto S, Kamel IR, et al. Distinction of long bone stress fractures from pathologic fractures on cross-sectional imaging: how successful are we? AJR Am J Roentgenol 2005;185(4):915–924

Phillips CD, Pope TL Jr, Jones JE, Keats TE, MacMillan RH III. Nontraumatic avulsion of the lesser trochanter: a pathognomonic sign of metastatic disease? Skeletal Radiol 1988;17(2):106–110

■ Case 70

Murphey MD, Robbin MR, McRae GA, Flemming DJ, Temple HT, Kransdorf MJ. The many faces of osteosarcoma. Radiographics 1997;17(5):1205–1231

Murphey MD, wan Jaovisidha S, Temple HT, Gannon FH, Jelinek JS, Malawer MM. Telangiectatic osteosarcoma: radiologic-pathologic comparison. Radiology 2003;229(2):545–553

White LM, Kandel R. Osteoid-producing tumors of bone. Semin Musculoskelet Radiol 2000;4(1):25–43

■ Case 71

Cobby MJ, Schweitzer ME, Resnick D. The deep lateral femoral notch: an indirect sign of a torn anterior cruciate ligament. Radiology 1992;184(3):855–858

Pao DG. The lateral femoral notch sign. Radiology 2001;219(3):800–801

Sanders TG, Medynski MA, Feller JF, Lawhorn KW. Bone contusion patterns of the knee at MR imaging: footprint of the mechanism of injury. Radiographics 2000;20(Spec No):S135–S151

■ Case 72

Chaudhary SB, Hullinger H, Vives MJ. Management of acute spinal fractures in ankylosing spondylitis. ISRN Rheumatol 2011;2011:150484

Jacobson JA, Girish G, Jiang Y, Resnick D. Radiographic evaluation of arthritis: inflammatory conditions. Radiology 2008;248(2):378–389

Wang YF, Teng MM, Chang CY, Wu HT, Wang ST. Imaging manifestations of spinal fractures in ankylosing spondylitis. AJNR Am J Neuroradiol 2005;26(8):2067–2076

■ **Case 73**

May DA, Disler DG, Jones EA, Balkissoon AA, Manaster BJ. Abnormal signal intensity in skeletal muscle at MR imaging: patterns, pearls, and pitfalls. Radiographics 2000;20(Spec No):S295–S315

Schulze M, Kötter I, Ernemann U, et al. MRI findings in inflammatory muscle diseases and their noninflammatory mimics. AJR Am J Roentgenol 2009;192(6):1708–1716

■ **Case 74**

Collins J. Chest wall trauma. J Thorac Imaging 2000;15(2):112–119

Kreeger MC, Bhargava P. Case 162: scapulothoracic dissociation. Radiology 2010;257(1):290–293

Miller LA. Chest wall, lung, and pleural space trauma. Radiol Clin North Am 2006;44(2):213–224, viii

■ **Case 75**

Bennett DL, Ohashi K, El-Khoury GY. Spondyloarthropathies: ankylosing spondylitis and psoriatic arthritis. Radiol Clin North Am 2004;42(1):121–134

Jacobson JA, Girish G, Jiang Y, Resnick D. Radiographic evaluation of arthritis: inflammatory conditions. Radiology 2008;248(2):378–389

■ **Case 76**

Chew FS, Ramsdell MG, Keel SB. Metallosis after total knee replacement. AJR Am J Roentgenol 1998;170(6):1556

Fritz J, Lurie B, Miller TT, Potter HG. MR imaging of hip arthroplasty implants. Radiographics 2014;34(4):E106–E132

Heffernan EJ, Alkubaidan FO, Nielsen TO, Munk PL. The imaging appearances of metallosis. Skeletal Radiol 2008;37(1):59–62

Keogh CF, Munk PL, Gee R, Chan LP, Marchinkow LO. Imaging of the painful hip arthroplasty. AJR Am J Roentgenol 2003;180(1):115–120

Llauger J, Palmer J, Rosón N, Bagué S, Camins A, Cremades R. Nonseptic monoarthritis: imaging features with clinical and histopathologic correlation. Radiographics 2000;20(Spec No):S263–S278

■ **Case 77**

Floemer F, Morrison WB, Bongartz G, Ledermann HP. MRI characteristics of olecranon bursitis. AJR Am J Roentgenol 2004;183(1):29–34

■ **Case 78**

Babini JC, Gusis SE, Babini SM, Cocco JA. Superolateral erosions of the humeral head in chronic inflammatory arthropathies. Skeletal Radiol 1992;21(8):515–517

Jacobson JA, Girish G, Jiang Y, Resnick D. Radiographic evaluation of arthritis: inflammatory conditions. Radiology 2008;248(2):378–389

■ **Case 79**

Anderson MW, Greenspan A. Stress fractures. Radiology 1996;199(1):1–12

Daffner RH, Pavlov H. Stress fractures: current concepts. AJR Am J Roentgenol 1992;159(2):245–252

■ **Case 80**

Jacobson JA, Girish G, Jiang Y, Resnick D. Radiographic evaluation of arthritis: inflammatory conditions. Radiology 2008;248(2):378–389

Sommer OJ, Kladosek A, Weiler V, Czembirek H, Boeck M, Stiskal M. Rheumatoid arthritis: a practical guide to state-of-the-art imaging, image interpretation, and clinical implications. Radiographics 2005;25(2):381–398

■ **Case 81**

Campagna R, Pessis E, Biau DJ, et al. Is superolateral Hoffa fat pad edema a consequence of impingement between lateral femoral condyle and patellar ligament? Radiology 2012;263(2):469–474

Diederichs G, Issever AS, Scheffler S. MR imaging of patellar instability: injury patterns and assessment of risk factors. Radiographics 2010;30(4):961–981

■ Case 82

Andrews CL. From the RSNA Refresher Courses. Radiological Society of North America. Evaluation of the marrow space in the adult hip. Radiographics 2000;20(Spec No):S27–S42

Korompilias AV, Karantanas AH, Lykissas MG, Beris AE. Bone marrow edema syndrome. Skeletal Radiol 2009;38(5):425–436

Manaster BJ. From the RSNA Refresher Courses. Radiological Society of North America. Adult chronic hip pain: radiographic evaluation. Radiographics 2000;20(Spec No):S3–S25

Vande Berg BE, Malghem JJ, Labaisse MA, Noel HM, Maldague BE. MR imaging of avascular necrosis and transient marrow edema of the femoral head. Radiographics 1993;13(3):501–520

■ Case 83

Jacobson JA, Girish G, Jiang Y, Sabb BJ. Radiographic evaluation of arthritis: degenerative joint disease and variations. Radiology 2008;248(3):737–747

Steinbach LS. Calcium pyrophosphate dihydrate and calcium hydroxyapatite crystal deposition diseases: imaging perspectives. Radiol Clin North Am 2004;42(1):185–205, vii

■ Case 84

Ashman CJ, Klecker RJ, Yu JS. Forefoot pain involving the metatarsal region: differential diagnosis with MR imaging. Radiographics 2001;21(6):1425–1440

Harty MP. Imaging of pediatric foot disorders. Radiol Clin North Am 2001;39(4):733–748

Torriani M, Thomas BJ, Bredella MA, Ouellette H. MRI of metatarsal head subchondral fractures in patients with forefoot pain. AJR Am J Roentgenol 2008;190(3):570–575

■ Case 85

Llauger J, Palmer J, Rosón N, Cremades R, Bagué S. Pigmented villonodular synovitis and giant cell tumors of the tendon sheath: radiologic and pathologic features. AJR Am J Roentgenol 1999;172(4):1087–1091

Murphey MD, Rhee JH, Lewis RB, Fanburg-Smith JC, Flemming DJ, Walker EA. Pigmented villonodular synovitis: radiologic-pathologic correlation. Radiographics 2008;28(5):1493–1518

Sheldon PJ, Forrester DM, Learch TJ. Imaging of intraarticular masses. Radiographics 2005;25(1):105–119

■ Case 86

Cothran RL Jr, Helms C. Quadrilateral space syndrome: incidence of imaging findings in a population referred for MRI of the shoulder. AJR Am J Roentgenol 2005;184(3):989–992

Robinson P, White LM, Lax M, Salonen D, Bell RS. Quadrilateral space syndrome caused by glenoid labral cyst. AJR Am J Roentgenol 2000;175(4):1103–1105

Yanny S, Toms AP. MR patterns of denervation around the shoulder. AJR Am J Roentgenol 2010;195(2):W157–W163

■ Case 87

Palmer WE. Femoroacetabular impingement: caution is warranted in making imaging-based assumptions and diagnoses. Radiology 2010;257(1):4–7

Tannast M, Siebenrock KA, Anderson SE. Femoroacetabular impingement: radiographic diagnosis—what the radiologist should know. AJR Am J Roentgenol 2007;188(6):1540–1552

■ Case 88

Donovan A, Schweitzer ME. Use of MR imaging in diagnosing diabetes-related pedal osteomyelitis. Radiographics 2010;30(3):723–736

Jones EA, Manaster BJ, May DA, Disler DG. Neuropathic osteoarthropathy: diagnostic dilemmas and differential diagnosis. Radiographics 2000;20(Spec No):S279–S293

■ Case 89

Iyer RS, Chapman T, Chew FS. Pediatric bone imaging: diagnostic imaging of osteoid osteoma. AJR Am J Roentgenol 2012;198(5):1039–1052

Kransdorf MJ, Stull MA, Gilkey FW, Moser RP Jr. Osteoid osteoma. Radiographics 1991;11(4):671–696

■ Case 90

Greenspan A, Tehranzadeh J. Imaging of infectious arthritis. Radiol Clin North Am 2001;39(2):267–276

Jacobson JA, Girish G, Jiang Y, Resnick D. Radiographic evaluation of arthritis: inflammatory conditions. Radiology 2008;248(2):378–389

Karchevsky M, Schweitzer ME, Morrison WB, Parellada JA. MRI findings of septic arthritis and associated osteomyelitis in adults. AJR Am J Roentgenol 2004;182(1):119–122

■ Case 91

Chew FS. Radiology of the hands: review and self-assessment module. AJR Am J Roentgenol 2005; 184(6, Suppl):S157–S168

Greenspan A. Erosive osteoarthritis. Semin Musculoskelet Radiol 2003;7(2):155–159

■ Case 92

Dupuis CS, Westra SJ, Makris J, Wallace EC. Injuries and conditions of the extensor mechanism of the pediatric knee. Radiographics 2009;29(3):877–886

■ Case 93

Hong SH, Choi JY, Lee JW, Kim NR, Choi JA, Kang HS. MR imaging assessment of the spine: infection or an imitation? Radiographics 2009;29(2):599–612

Varma R, Lander P, Assaf A. Imaging of pyogenic infectious spondylodiskitis. Radiol Clin North Am 2001;39(2):203–213

■ Case 94

Murphey MD, Choi JJ, Kransdorf MJ, Flemming DJ, Gannon FH. Imaging of osteochondroma: variants and complications with radiologic-pathologic correlation. Radiographics 2000;20(5):1407–1434

■ Case 95

O'Regan KN, Jagannathan J, Krajewski K, et al. Imaging of liposarcoma: classification, patterns of tumor recurrence, and response to treatment. AJR Am J Roentgenol 2011;197(1):W37–W43

Sung MS, Kang HS, Suh JS, et al. Myxoid liposarcoma: appearance at MR imaging with histologic correlation. Radiographics 2000;20(4):1007–1019

■ Case 96

Mulcahy H, Chew FS. Current concepts of hip arthroplasty for radiologists: part 2, revisions and complications. AJR Am J Roentgenol 2012;199(3):570–580

Nicolaou S, Liang T, Murphy DT, Korzan JR, Ouellette H, Munk P. Dual-energy CT: a promising new technique for assessment of the musculoskeletal system. AJR Am J Roentgenol 2012;199(5, Suppl):S78–S86

Roth TD, Maertz NA, Parr JA, Buckwalter KA, Choplin RH. CT of the hip prosthesis: appearance of components, fixation, and complications. Radiographics 2012;32(4):1089–1107

■ Case 97

Bernard SA, Murphey MD, Flemming DJ, Kransdorf MJ. Improved differentiation of benign osteochondromas from secondary chondrosarcomas with standardized measurement of cartilage cap at CT and MR imaging. Radiology 2010;255(3):857–865

Douis H, Saifuddin A. The imaging of cartilaginous bone tumours. II. Chondrosarcoma. Skeletal Radiol 2013;42(5):611–626

■ Case 98

Dong Q, Fessell DP. Achilles tendon ultrasound technique. AJR Am J Roentgenol 2009;193(3):W173

Rosenberg ZS, Beltran J, Bencardino JT. MR imaging of the ankle and foot. Radiographics 2000;20(Spec No):S153–S179

Schweitzer ME, Karasick D. MR imaging of disorders of the Achilles tendon. AJR Am J Roentgenol 2000;175(3):613–625

Zbojniewicz AM. US for diagnosis of musculoskeletal conditions in the young athlete: emphasis on dynamic assessment. Radiographics 2014;34(5):1145–1162

■ **Case 99**

Sookur PA, Naraghi AM, Bleakney RR, Jalan R, Chan O, White LM. Accessory muscles: anatomy, symptoms, and radiologic evaluation. Radiographics 2008;28(2):481–499

Wang XT, Rosenberg ZS, Mechlin MB, Schweitzer ME. Normal variants and diseases of the peroneal tendons and superior peroneal retinaculum: MR imaging features. Radiographics 2005;25(3):587–602

■ **Case 100**

Mohankumar R, Palisch A, Khan W, White LM, Morrison WB. Meniscal ossicle: posttraumatic origin and association with posterior meniscal root tears. AJR Am J Roentgenol 2014;203(5):1040–1046

Index

Locators refer to case number. Locators in boldface indicate primary diagnosis.